MRCP PACES
Ethics and Communication Skills

Iqbal Khan BSc, PhD, MRCP (UK)
Specialist Registrar in Gastroenterology
University Hospital, Birmingham

Radcliffe Publishing
Oxford • Seattle

Radcliffe Publishing Ltd
18 Marcham Road
Abingdon
Oxon OX14 1AA
United Kingdom

www.radcliffe-oxford.com
Electronic catalogue and worldwide online ordering facility.

British Library Cataloguing in Publication Data

A catalogue record for this book is available from the British Library.

ISBN-10 1 85775 753 X
ISBN-13 978 1 85775 753 8

Typeset by Anne Joshua & Associates, Oxford, UK
Printed and bound by TJ International Ltd, Padstow, Cornwall

I dedicate this book to my wife Nuzhat, without whose encouragement this book would not have been possible.

Contents

Preface

The Royal College of Physicians (RCP) introduced the Practical Assessment of Clinical Examination Skills (PACES) exam in June 2001. With it they introduced a station that is very relevant to the day-to-day practice of medicine. This station is based around a candidate's understanding of ethical issues and their ability to communicate effectively with the patient, relative or colleagues.

The problem for the candidates is that in most medical schools, students receive little formal training in ethics and communication skills (although the situation does seem to be changing in the UK) and naturally find the station very difficult, and often fail because of it. This situation is not helped by the fact that busy junior doctors working in busy hospitals often cannot afford the time to delve through volumes of material to try and pass this station and instead focus on the clinical stations.

This concise text has been prepared with those busy junior doctors in mind. It is intentionally not long-winded and I hope will get you *up to speed* relatively quickly. I should say that it is not intended as a comprehensive collection of all the possible scenarios that may arise, but instead its aim is to introduce you to the sorts of scenario you are likely to meet in the exam and give you some scope for practice. This in turn will hopefully help you pass the exam and go some way towards helping you with your medical career.

It is strongly recommend that during the weeks and months leading up to the *big day*, you try and spend as much time as possible in practising role-play with your colleagues/friends in front of the mirror or even with the cat (I'm sure it is impossible for junior doctors to keep a dog!). Some people find the use of videoing in role-play very useful. Others find that it is a good way to destroy their confidence.

At this point I should like to emphasise that all the cases in this book, the names of doctors, patients and relatives are fictitious and any similarity to real people and events is by coincidence.
Good luck!

Iqbal Khan
January 2006
Iqbalkhan@doctors.org.uk

About the author

Iqbal Khan is a specialist registrar in gastroenterology and general internal medicine on the West Midlands Rotation. He was born in Birmingham and studied at the University of Sheffield. After obtaining a dual honours degree in biochemistry and physiology, he went on to study medicine. He also conducted research with an enthusiastic gastroenterologist for a PhD, and it was this experience that initiated his interest in gastroenterology.

Over the years he has helped many senior house officers to get through their MRCP exams and medical students to get through their finals and strongly believes that the best way to learn is by teaching others.

How to use this book

This book is designed to provide busy doctors with common case scenarios, which they can use to practise and develop their communication skills for the PACES exam. Moreover, this book should provide a useful introduction to basic medical ethics. It is suggested that two or more people work together to practise the cases provided. One of the team can act as the exam candidate and should only be provided with the information given as the *scenario*. Another can act as the surrogate patient/relative. It is best to think through the roles and try to make the situation as realistic as possible. Hence, they are best practised in a quiet, bleep-free environment.

Work through each case following the format of the exam:

- Spend 2 minutes reading through the case and mentally preparing for the case.
- The discussion should take 14 minutes.
- Allow 1 minute for reflection.
- The examiners have 5 minutes to question you on the case.
- Total time for each case is 22 minutes (20 minutes in the exam room).

Each case begins with a description of the scenario. This is very similar to that which will be encountered in the exam itself. The candidate must read this and not have access to the rest of the text. The individual acting as the subject/patient can review the case and see their individual information. The prompts are suggested questions that the subject may use on the candidate. It is perfectly OK not to use any of them, but I have included them to help the discussion to flow, particularly if you are practising the case with a non-medical person (spouse, parents, etc.).

Once a case has been conducted, the discussion and ethical issues can be reviewed. This always includes a 'possible interview plan' and other relevant issues. The possible interview plan is exactly that. It is one possible plan that you can follow while having the discussion; you may even come to the conclusion that it isn't the best possible plan. There are infinite permutations any 14-minute medical discussion can follow and it depends upon a number of variables. These include the medical facts available and the individual's communication and linguistic skills. Once you start to acquire the relevant knowledge on ethical and NHS issues, and develop communication skills, you will start to see the patterns in the cases and feel confident that you could tackle similar cases presented to you in the exam itself.

By the time you have come to study for the PACES exam, it will have become apparent that much of the MRCP exam follows a format where pattern recognition is the key to success. This is also true for the PACES exam, including the 'ethics and communication skills' station. Practise and you will succeed.

Chapter 1

Basic medical ethics

Ethical theory

Along with scientific knowledge, moral issues and value judgements have always been a very important part of medical practice. Over the last 250 years these issues have been analysed and two fundamental theories on medical ethics have been particularly influential in Western medicine:

1 **Consequentialism (utilitarianism):** Simplified, this asks for the consequences of each action to be addressed and that with the foreseeable most favourable consequence is the best path to follow. The most favourable consequence is one where there is the least human suffering and the most happiness.

2 **Duty-based ethics (deontological):** This theory dictates that we are duty-bound to certain actions in our medical practice irrespective of the consequences. For instance, it is important to always be honest with our patients. In contrast, a utilitarian may argue that it is better to lie to a terminally ill patient about their prognosis if the truth is likely to add to their suffering.

In real life, often the two theories coexist in medical practice. For instance, it is often important that we tell the patient the truth about a terminal diagnosis. However, we may not be absolutely frank about their prognosis. I've often heard colleagues, when directly challenged, say things like, '. . . I'm sorry I don't have a crystal ball that tells me the future', or even, 'Well how long is a piece of string?'

Most doctors, although oblivious to moral theories, do recognise that there are some basic *principles* of medical ethics that are important to our practice. The four principles that are most well recognised and used are:

1   *Autonomy.* Autonomy means self-rule, and this principle urges healthcare providers to respect the patient's wishes and decisions, even if they are felt to be wrong.
2   *Beneficence.* Literally this means doing good, and promotes the doctor to act in the patient's best interest.
3   *Non-maleficence.* To do no harm, even if we are unable to do good.
4   *Justice.* To treat all patients equally and thus to give medical resources equally.

Patient consent

In English law the legal position is said to adopt the famous statement of Judge Cardozo:

> Every human being of adult years and sound mind has the right to determine what shall be done with his own body; and a surgeon who performs an operation without his patient's consent commits an assault [sic. battery] for which he is liable in damages.

Valid consent depends on the premises that a doctor has disclosed all relevant information to a *competent* patient, and that the patient understands this information and makes the appropriate decision voluntarily. This should not be confused with *assent*, which is mere submission by the patient to the doctor's authoritative order (Faden and Beauchamp, 1986). Under English law, patients can sue their doctor for *battery* (any intentional non-consensual contact) if a procedure has been performed without proper consent. Moreover, a doctor may be found *negligent* if a procedure is performed without disclosing all the relevant information.

Competence (or in legal jargon, 'to have capacity')

Any competent patient over 18 years old (16 years in Scotland) can refuse treatment, *even if it is likely to be life-saving.* When patients are thought to be incompetent, the doctor should act in the best interest of the patient, according to their professional judgement. The Bolam test (i.e. a reasonable body of medical opinion would support the actions of the doctor) can be applied in this situation. Under English law, there is no proxy consent for an incompetent individual by family or friends, although they may provide valuable information. Some important issues to assess a patient's competence or capacity are:

- a patient should not be deemed incompetent just because they make an imprudent or unwise decision
- a patient does not have to be globally competent to provide valid consent. It is simply adequate that they understand the principles surrounding the procedure to be performed
- when assessing capacity, simply look at the 'balance of probabilities' of a patient being competent, as opposed to 'beyond reasonable doubt', which is applied in criminal cases.

Patients are thought to have capacity if they are able to:

- comprehend and retain information relevant to making the decision
- believe this information
- weigh the information and make a decision.

It is presumed that 16–17-year-olds have capacity to give consent, unless the contrary has been shown. Patients under 16 years of age are not presumed to have capacity unless they satisfy health professionals to the contrary. These patients are then termed 'Gillick competent', following the landmark case – *Gillick* v *West Norfolk and Wisbebech AHA and DHSS* (1985) (*see* landmark case p. 6) Generally, parents are obliged to act in the patient's best interest and to provide consent.

Form of consent

Consent is fundamentally a state of mind, where the patient submits to the proposed treatment. The two recognised forms of consent are 'express' and 'implied'. The patient may explicitly agree to a form of treatment either orally or in writing, for example when signing a consent form for a surgical procedure. In this situation the consent is said to be express. During routine clinical practice, most consent is implied because of the patient's conduct. For instance, if you wish to insert a venous cannulae into the back of a patient's hand and the patient holds out his hand, clearly the patient consents to the procedure. The scope of implied consent should not be too widely construed. For instance, if a patient enters a room for a clinic visit, s/he has only consented to the consultation and not necessarily to a physical examination.

Lawful treatment without consent

The House of Lords previously (1989) addressed the issue of treating patients who were unable to give consent either because they lacked capacity or had become incapacitated (for example because of illness or general anaesthesia). They concluded:

> In common law a doctor can lawfully operate on or give other treatment to adult patients who are incapable of consenting to his doing so, provided that the operation or treatment is in the best interest of such patients. The operation will be in their best interests only if it is carried out in order either to save their lives or to ensure improvement or prevent deterioration in their physical or mental health.

'Common law' (also known as the 'adversarial system') originally developed in historical England from judicial decisions that were based in tradition, custom and precedent. The form of reasoning used in common law is known as 'case-based reasoning' or 'casuistry'. The common law was devised as a means of compensating someone for wrongful acts known as 'torts', including both intentional torts and torts caused by negligence. It also served as a body of law recognising and regulating contracts. Common law may be unwritten or written in statutes or codes.

Treating patients in their 'best interest' gives doctors the ability to institute a broad range of interventions, particularly in emergency settings.

Veracity

Truthfulness is fundamental to the trust the patient has in their doctor and consent based on deceit and inaccurate information is not valid. This is particularly true if the 'informed consent' is carried out as a ritual to protect against later liability. 'Therapeutic privilege' is an exception to this rule and refers to information, which may have been withheld from a patient because it was felt to be detrimental to their wellbeing. Generally speaking, honesty is the best policy.

Advance directive (living will)

This is a formally written and witnessed statement a competent person may make regarding treatment they should like to receive if they were to become incompetent. For example, a patient with motor neurone disease may state that they do not want to be resuscitated in the event of a cardiac arrest when they are severely debilitated and unable to communicate.

LANDMARK CASE

Sidaway 1984

Mrs Sidaway had presented to a neurosurgeon with recurrent pain in her neck and shoulders, which was thought to be due to nerve root compression. An operation was subsequently undertaken to release the roots, which unfortunately left Mrs Sidaway with partial paralysis. The risk of this occurring was 1–2 per cent, even in the hands of a skilled surgeon. Mrs Sidaway went on to sue the hospital arguing that she would not have given consent to the procedure if she had been told about the possibility of this outcome, and as such her surgeon had been negligent. The Bolam test was applied at court and Mrs Sidaway lost the case. The evidence before the court was that a responsible body of opinion would consider the risk of paralysis small enough not to be presented to the patient.

LANDMARK CASE

Re C (Adult refusal to medical treatment)

C was a chronic schizophrenic and an inmate at Broadmoor Hospital. He developed gangrene in his right foot and medical opinion was that his leg should be amputated. C refused to give consent and the case went to court. The judge was satisfied that although C lacked general capacity, he did have sufficient insight to refuse the amputation. This case laid down the three stages by which a court could determine a patient's capacity, i.e.:

1   Comprehend and retain information
2   Believe it
3   Weigh it in the balance and arrive at a choice

LANDMARK CASE

Gillick v West Norfolk and Wisbebech AHA and DHSS (1985)

The concept of Gillick competence came about following this case where the central issue was the right of a doctor to prescribe contraception to a girl under the age of 16 years without parental consent. During the hearing Lord Scarman commented that, '. . . as a matter of law the parental right to determine whether or not their minor child below the age of 16 will have medical treatment terminates if and when the child achieves sufficient understanding and intelligence to enable him to understand fully what is proposed'. Hence children of any age can consent to or refuse treatment if they are deemed Gillick competent by a court of law.

Confidentiality

Confidentiality is the cornerstone of the doctor–patient relationship, and it supports the principle of patient autonomy, which emphasises the patient's right to control over their life. The legal aspects of confidentiality lie in common law. This basically dictates that a doctor is obliged to maintain patient confidentiality except under situations where it is of greater public interest. Note that this may only be one member of the public! Examples of situations where a doctor *must* breach confidentiality include:

- births and deaths [Births and Deaths Registration Act 1953]
- notifiable diseases [Notifiable Diseases Act 1984]
- drug addiction [Misuse of Drugs Act 1973]
- under court orders
- details of a driver alleged to be guilty under the Road Traffic Act [1988] to the police.

There are certain situations where a doctor has the *discretion* to breach confidentiality (these are probably those that are more likely to feature in the PACES exam). Such situations include:

- where there is a third party at significant risk of harm, for example the partner of an HIV-positive patient
- a driver known to be an uncontrolled epileptic who continues to drive
- sharing information with other healthcare workers in the interest of the patient.

It is important to realise that the obligation to keep information confidential applies even after the patient's death.

The Access to Health Records Act (1990) gives patients the general right to see their medical records, have them explained and obtain copies of them. If any of the information is inaccurate, the patient has the right to ask to have this changed.

LANDMARK CASE

X v Y 1988

The employees of a health authority divulged the names of two practising doctors who were being treated for HIV disease to a national newspaper. Publication of the details of the doctors involved was prevented when a judge decided that the public interest in maintaining confidentiality was greater than the public interest in making public the names of doctors who were practising medicine while known to be HIV positive.

Medical negligence

All doctors practising medicine need to be aware of the laws governing medical negligence. In cases where medical negligence is alleged the plaintiff must prove three separate points:

1 *Duty of care* is owed to them. This usually means that the defendant was the patient's hospital physician or general practitioner.
2 *A breach of the duty of care* has occurred.
3 *Damage* has occurred as a result of the breach.

If these three points can be proven then the 'Bolitho principle' applies and the defendant has been found negligent. In the UK, negligence was traditionally judged using the 'Bolam test' (*Bolam v Friern Hospital Management Committee (1957)*) (*see* landmark case p. 9). According to the Bolam test a doctor is not negligent if they have acted in accordance with a practice accepted as proper by a responsible body of medical opinion. This principle, however, has been perceived as being excessively reliant upon medical testimony supporting the defendant. In recent years there has been a shift from the traditional Bolam test because of the judgement given by the House of Lords in the case of Bolitho (*Bolitho v City and Hackney Health Authority (1997)*) (*see* landmark case p. 9). This ruling imposes a requirement that the standard being analysed must have considered the risks and benefits of competing options and hence the court's stance will be much more enquiring of the evidence offered by both parties. As the climate becomes increasingly litigious medical practitioners must have an understanding of this approach and the shift from the traditional Bolam test.

LANDMARK CASE

Bolam v *Friern Hospital Management Committee (1957)*

The Friern Hospital Management Committee was sued by Mr Bolam after his leg was broken during a course of electroconvulsive therapy (ECT). Mr Bolam argued that the doctors had been negligent by not providing a muscle relaxant during the ECT. During the subsequent trial it became apparent that while some practitioners felt it was necessary to give a muscle relaxant during ECT, others did not. Mr Bolam lost the case, as not giving a muscle relaxant was an acceptable practice. During the summing up of the case the judge proclaimed:

> *'A doctor is not guilty of negligence if he has acted in accordance with the practice accepted as proper by a responsible body of medical men skilled in that particular art. . . .'*

LANDMARK CASE

Bolitho v *City and Hackney Health Authority (1997)*

This is an important landmark case as it modified the Bolam result. A two-year-old child had been admitted to hospital with croup (after initially being discharged the day before with similar symptoms). Over the course of his admission he deteriorated to the extent that he had a cardiac arrest resulting in irreversible brain damage. A case of negligence was brought up against the paediatrics registrar who had been summoned three times, but failed to attend or send an appropriate deputy. The doctor was found to be clearly negligent in this respect. Hence it was established that the doctor had a duty of care and had breached this. It finally came to the point of whether this had resulted in damage and this is why this case is important. As there were eight expert witnesses called, five said that any competent doctor would have intubated the patient and the fact he wasn't intubated had resulted in the harm. However, the other three said that on the basis of the history it was responsible not to intubate the child and hence the outcome would have been the same. However, while there was a reasonable and responsible body of opinion in favour of the defendant, the judge still declared negligence as he felt that this opinion was not logical and 'not capable of withstanding logical analysis'. This is a subtle but significant change from the traditional Bolam test and establishes that it is a matter for the court and not medical opinion to establish the standard of professional care.

End-of-life decisions

End-of-life matters such as euthanasia, do-not-resuscitate orders and living wills have received much public attention and debate over the last few years. There has been great concern regarding doctors hastening death in patients who are terminally ill. Conversely, there are other people who are concerned that terminally ill patients are being kept alive 'artificially', hence prolonging their suffering. There are no easy solutions here and the debates will continue long into the night.

Euthanasia

This comes from the Greek, meaning 'a good death'. It can be further broken down into the following categories:

- *Active euthanasia.* The doctor performs an action that leads to the patient's death.

- *Passive euthanasia.* The doctor withholds or withdraws life-prolonging treatment leading to the patient's death.
- *Voluntary euthanasia.* The patient requests death of the doctor. This is not the same as an assisted suicide, where the patient takes their own life.
- *Non-voluntary euthanasia.* The patient has not expressed an opinion, e.g. may be a newborn.
- *Involuntary euthanasia.* The doctor takes the patient's life against their wishes. This amounts to murder.

It is fair to say that in the UK most doctors probably practise passive euthanasia, where treatment may be withdrawn from a patient whose prognosis is futile.

Arguments against active euthanasia include:

1 Slippery slope effect. If active euthanasia were to be legalised then bit by bit it may lead to euthanasia in patients for whom it would be inappropriate. The practice would vary between hospitals/hospices, where some would be more active than others.
2 People may use it as a means of exploiting the dying.
3 There is no need for euthanasia in a society where we have excellent palliative care facilities. With drugs like opiate analgesics, strong antiemetics and laxatives no patient need suffer greatly.

Arguments for active euthanasia:

1 We live in a society where passive euthanasia is generally accepted. Some people believe that it is a small step from this to active euthanasia, which would further alleviate suffering.
2 Suicide is legal now and often rational. The people who are the most disabled are unable to take their own lives (viz. motor neurone disease sufferer Diane Pretty).
3 Dying people are often sedated to unconsciousness; some people would argue that this is no different from dying.

LANDMARK CASE

Diane Pretty

Diane Pretty was a terminally ill woman with motor neurone disease, which had been diagnosed in 1999. She was expected to die because of this condition. Mrs Pretty had argued that her husband should be legally allowed to assist her suicide at the time of her choosing. She applied first to the Director of Public Prosecutions (DPP) via a letter written to the Prime Minister, Mr Tony Blair. Her application was refused. She then fought her case through the High Court, the House of Lords and the European Court of Human Rights. Her appeal was rejected in all of these courts. The case received massive media coverage and public attention. Mrs Pretty eventually died in May 2002 at the age of 43 years.

LANDMARK CASE

Annie Lindsell

Annie Lindsell was a 41-year-old attractive and articulate woman who previously had a very active life as an air hostess and actress. This all changed when she was diagnosed with motor neurone disease and she spent the final years of her life campaigning for a change in the UK law to allow assistance in dying. Not only did she give numerous interviews, but also addressed Parliament in 1996. The same year she had launched a legal case where she demanded reassurance that when she was terminally ill, 'brave' doctors would be able to administer treatments to palliate her effectively, even at the cost of shortening her life. She was particularly concerned about choking to death, which she had described as like 'living in a coffin'. It was felt that symptom control of terminally ill patients was ethically and legally permissible and her case was dismissed. She died naturally in 1997.

LANDMARK CASE:

Dr David Moor

Dr Moor, who died in 2000, worked as a GP in North-umberland. He had long been a supporter of euthanasia and in 1997 in interviews for radio, television and the newspapers he openly admitted to helping many terminally ill patients, over a 30-year period, to die by administering fatal doses of diamorphine. Dr Moor admitted in the interview that he had probably broken the law. The police subsequently charged him with the murder of George Liddell, an 85-year-old man with advanced cancer. Dr Moor was acquitted in May 1999. This landmark case emphasised the importance of the primary intention, i.e the diamorphine was administered to relieve pain and not to hasten death.

Do-not-resuscitate (DNR) orders

The British Medical Association (BMA), the Resuscitation Council (UK) and the Royal College of Nursing (RCN) have issued guidelines regarding resuscitation decisions (2001). The guidelines essentially say that:

- timely support for patients and people close to them, and effective, sensitive communication are essential
- decisions must be based on the individual patient's circumstances and reviewed regularly
- sensitive advance discussion should always be encouraged, but not forced
- information about CPR (cardiopulmonary resuscitation) and the chances of a successful outcome needs to be realistic
- information about CPR policies should be displayed for patients and staff
- leaflets should be available for patients and people close to them, explaining CPR, how decisions are made and their involvement in decisions

- decisions about attempting CPR must be communicated effectively to relevant health professionals
- in emergencies, if no advance decision has been made or is known, CPR should be attempted unless the patient has refused CPR, the patient is clearly in the terminal phase of illness, or the burdens of the treatment outweigh the benefits
- competent patients should be involved in discussions about attempting CPR unless they indicate that they do not want to be
- where patients lack competence to participate, people close to them can be helpful in reflecting their views
- patients' rights under the Human Rights Act must be taken into account when making the decision
- neither patients nor relatives can demand treatment that the healthcare team judges to be inappropriate, but all efforts will be made to accommodate wishes and preferences
- in England, Wales and Northern Ireland, relatives and people close to the patient are not entitled in law to take healthcare decisions for the patient
- in Scotland, adults may appoint a healthcare proxy to give consent to medical treatment
- health professionals need to be aware of the law in relation to decision making for children and young people.

Kübler-Ross's Stages of Dying

Elizabeth Kübler-Ross's book *On Death and Dying* (1969) helped to popularise a characterisation of the process of grief as steps or stages through which the dying and, to some extent, those close to them ordinarily pass. While she was hardly the originator of the idea, her book has provided access to this useful tool for thousands of healthcare professionals. Used carefully, these stages can be helpful in recognising and responding to the psychological state and needs of those in grief.

A note of caution should be offered from the outset: you should avoid thinking of these 'Five Stages of Dying' as necessary elements in an inevitable sequence or as levels to be mastered.

The stage of acceptance is not a goal to be accomplished by means of the other steps. While patients tend to go through a series of stages, they may go back and forth, skip about or have periods where the stages seem to overlap, all according to their particular needs. With this in mind, it is helpful to think of grief as tending to approximate five stages:

1 *Denial* of death because they are unable to admit to themselves that the patient might die and/or they will suffer the loss death represents.
2 *Anger* by which the pain of loss is projected onto others.
3 *Bargaining,* which represents a last effort at overcoming death by 'earning' longer life.
4 *Depression:* when the full impact of imminent death strikes them.
5 *Acceptance:* when the grieving come to grips with the fact of the patient's death and make preparation for it.

These stages reflect the needs of the dying patient and others, and the devices they use to cope with them. It is most important for you to remember that the loss by death to and of the patient is probably the greatest loss those affected will ever experience. The prospect of death, then, will be the greatest crisis one can face. For most people, this crisis can be endured only with at least the temporary help of coping devices like those suggested by the stages.

There are, of course, other models for understanding this important process, which are well worth reading. One that deserves your special consideration is in the work of Backer, Hannon and Russell (Backer *et al.*, 1994).

Doctrine of double effect

This principle, which was developed in the Middle Ages by Roman Catholic theologians, is used to justify medical treatments; harm or death is a foreseen consequence. The doctrine applies if the desired outcome is judged to be 'good' (e.g. to relieve patient suffering) and the 'bad' outcome (e.g. the patient's death) is not intended. Hence it is ethically correct to administer opiate drugs to a terminally ill patient, even though it is likely to bring on their death. Some people find this doctrine seriously flawed as it offers the doctor a convenient evasion of responsibility and takes no account of the patient's wishes. As such, it violates the patient's provision of informed consent and the right of self-determination (Quill *et al.*, 1997).

Sanctity of life doctrine

The fundamental principle is that all human life has worth and should therefore be preserved, irrespective of the quality of that life. This principle is in keeping with the general perception of what doctors should do, which is to save and preserve life. The greatest challenge to this doctrine comes from the concept of quality of life as opposed to quantity. The question remains: Who defines the quality of life – the doctor, the patient, the family or perhaps the nurse? The answer is, of course, the patient, but we are back to 'square one', when the patient is unable to communicate their attitude.

Research ethics

'If you steal from one author it's plagiarism. If you steal from many it is research.'
(Wilson Mizner, in Alva Johnston's *The Legendary Mizners*)

Moral codes on the conduct of research involving human subjects have been developed to prevent appalling human abuse in the name of medical research. The best-recognised of these are the 'experiments' carried out on Jewish inmates in the Nazi concentration camps.

Codes of conduct

The Nuremberg Code was developed following the Nuremberg Trials for war criminals in 1948. It was a 10-point code designed to prevent future mistreatment of people in the name of research. In 1964 these principles were adopted by the 18th

World Medical Assembly and elaborated into The Declaration of Helsinki, so-called because the congress took place in that city. The Declaration of Helsinki has been revised on a number of occasions to incorporate new developments. The most recent revision was in the USA in 2002. The full declaration is a weighty document and not something to be committed to memory (you are certainly not required to know it for the PACES examination!). But some key excerpts are shown here:

Medical research involving human subjects includes research on identifiable human material or identifiable data.

In medical research on human subjects, considerations related to the well-being of the human subject should take precedence over the interests of science and society.

Medical research involving human subjects should only be conducted if the importance of the objective outweighs the inherent risks and burdens to the subject. This is especially important when the human subjects are healthy volunteers.

For a research subject who is legally incompetent, physically or mentally incapable of giving consent or is a legally incompetent minor, the investigator must obtain informed consent from the legally authorised representative in accordance with applicable law. These groups should not be included in research unless the research is necessary to promote the health of the population represented and this research cannot instead be performed on legally competent persons.

The subjects must be volunteers and informed participants in the research project.

The physician should fully inform the patient which aspects of the care are related to the research. The refusal of a patient to participate in a study must never interfere with the patient–physician relationship.

The ethics committee

The Department of Health (DoH) requires district health authorities to set up local research and ethics committees (LREC). If more than five LRECs are involved in a research project, a multicentre research ethics committee (MREC) needs to be involved. There is no legal requirement for potential researchers to submit projects to the LREC. However, most funding bodies will not give awards without LREC approval for a project. In addition, without approval, access to NHS patients and their notes would be denied.

The General Medical Council (GMC)

The General Medical Council (GMC) is a registered charity, which was established under the Medical Act of 1858 to protect the interest of the patients. However, it has been accused of protecting the interest of the doctor. The Council itself is made up of 35 members, who include doctors, lay people and academics. The only official register of all the doctors practising in the UK is kept by the GMC.

The GMC has produced several publications to advise doctors. These can be accessed on the GMC website (www.gmc-uk.org/index.htm). The following essential duties of a doctor are promoted by the GMC:

- make the care of your patient your first concern
- treat every patient politely and considerately
- respect patients' dignity and privacy
- listen to patients and respect their views
- give patients information in a way they can understand
- respect the rights of patients to be fully involved in decisions about their care
- keep your professional knowledge and skills up to date
- recognise the limits of your professional competence
- be honest and trustworthy
- respect and protect confidential information
- make sure that your personal beliefs do not prejudice your patients' care
- act quickly to protect patients from risk if you have good reason to believe that you or a colleague may not be fit to practise

- avoid abusing your position as a doctor
- work with colleagues in the ways that best serve patients' interests.

Whistle blowing

As the above list shows, the GMC encourages doctors to act if they feel that a colleague is not fit to practise. In its guidelines it is particularly keen for a doctor to be referred to the GMC under the following circumstances:

- local action would not be practical
- you have tried local action and it has failed
- the problem is so serious that we clearly need to be involved, or
- the doctor has been convicted of a criminal offence.

LANDMARK CASE

The Bristol heart deaths

This scandal centred on paediatric heart surgery at the Bristol Royal Infirmary. An anaesthetist (Dr Stephen Bolsin) alleged that there was a major problem with the mortality rates of the paediatric heart surgeons working at the Infirmary. His voice was largely ignored and the surgeons continued to operate. Eventually an independent enquiry was launched in 1995 and the GMC carried out an investigation in 1998. It investigated 53 operations and the results showed that 29 children had died and four had suffered brain damage. One of the surgeons (Mr James Wisheart) and the chief executive (Dr John Roylance) were struck off, while another surgeon (Mr Janardan Dhasmana) was banned from operating on children for three years. The subsequent Bristol public enquiry was the largest-ever independent investigation into clinical practice in the NHS.

LANDMARK CASE

The Alder Hey scandal

During the Bristol Enquiry, Professor Robert Anderson, of Great Ormond Street Hospital, London, reported that the largest UK organ collection was at Alder Hey Children's Hospital, Liverpool. The Health Secretary, Frank Dobson, ordered a national inquiry. This confirmed that a huge collection of organs had been built up at the hospital without the consent of parents. Professor van Velzen, pathologist, was particularly criticised and was suspended as it was reported that during his tenure, the size of the collection had grown rapidly while the standard of postmortem examinations declined to unacceptable standards. Professor van Velzen was suspended. The subsequent Alder Hey Report recommended that organs beyond those establishing cause of death should not be retained unless consent has been properly obtained. It was also suggested that the Human Tissue Act 2004 should be amended to make 'a failure to obtain fully informed consent' a criminal offence.

LANDMARK CASE

Harold Shipman

This GP from Manchester was convicted in 2000 of the murders of 15 elderly women in his care. Subsequent enquiries have suggested that he may have been responsible for the deaths of several hundred people (predominately elderly women). The GMC struck Dr Shipman off the medical register, but the case had achieved immense public notoriety and had a serious long-term effect on the public's faith in doctors.

Communication skills

It is accepted that good communication skills are essential to effective medical practice and, as such, are becoming an integral part of the medical curriculum and quite correctly are now tested during the PACES exam. Communication is important not only in the context of doctor–patient (or family members) interaction, but also between healthcare professionals. The benefits to the patient are obvious as effective communication gives them better insight into their conditions and may aid compliance and quality of life. Less well cited, but perhaps just as important, are the advantages to the doctors. Medicine is an emotionally demanding profession and effective communication skills may relieve doctors of some of the pressures of dealing with the difficult situations. Poor communication with patients is thought to contribute to psychological morbidity, low personal achievement and emotional burnout. Competent communication enhances job satisfaction and the satisfaction of patients, who are less likely to complain or sue.

Can you learn communication skills?

There is no doubt that some people are inherently better at communicating than others. They are not necessarily better doctors, but are perhaps more likely to pass the PACES exam as they demonstrate better communication skills when at stations 2 and 4 and will be more effective at communicating their ideas to the examiners. For the others there are two possible causes for their comparatively poor communication skills. First, the problem is a perceived one and they are actually better communicators than they will give themself credit for. It's a matter of practice to enhance self-confidence. I hope the following chapter in this book will give scope for practice. The second possibility is that they genuinely lack the skills of an effective communicator. This is something that cannot be remedied 'overnight' and healthcare professionals generally spend their lives improving these skills. However, there is evidence (Maguire *et al.*, 1989) that effective communication skills can be learnt or improved. The best way to do this is by practice and feedback. The feedback on your communication skills can come back from other colleagues (ideally seniors), patients and even yourself with the use of video recording.

Important factors

There are three factors that contribute to the interaction between the doctor and the patient. These include, the interview setting, the patient-related factors and the doctor-related factors.

Factor 1: The interview setting

Generally it is important that there is privacy. It is hard for people to express emotions if there are third parties present. At the PACES station there will be at least two examiners present, so the privacy will have to be imagined. Other important factors include comfortable surroundings (not in your control!) and seating arrangements. It's recognised that doctor and patient seating arrangements affect communication. For instance, communication is hindered if doctor and patient sit opposite each other across a desk and helped if they sit close to one another where the patient feels at ease and visual cues are easier to pick up. The seating in the interview room will be in place and the examiners are unlikely to appreciate you moving the furniture. However, they will not mind subtle movement of chairs to aid communication.

Factor 2: Patient-related factors

The patient's character and past experiences have a profound effect on how they communicate with doctors. Particularly important are psychological factors such as anger and denial and physical symptoms of the illness. Hence all patients cannot be treated the same and your approach needs to be suited to that individual patient.

Factor 3: Doctor-related factors

It is very important to realise that your own personal experiences and individual characteristics have an important bearing upon how you deal with an individual patient.

The interview

Beginning

Confirm the patient's identity, greet them by name and, if appropriate, shake their hand while introducing yourself. Explain the purpose of the interview.

Middle

Maintain good eye contact and attentive listening, and appear sympathetic. Be alert and responsive to verbal and nonverbal cues. Ask more open questions at the beginning and closed and specific questions as facts are ascertained. When appropriate, clarify what the patient has told you and build on it. Let the patient talk as long as it is relevant. Avoid interrupting the patient and don't ask overcomplicated questions.

End

Summarise and confirm the facts with the patient. Ensure there is a follow-up plan. Thank the patient.

It is important that the interview is entirely *purposeful.* The questions should not be simply conversational or leading, but should be probing and relevant. It is important that you listen to the patient and at least seem to be very attentive. Rapport is better and patients are more forthcoming with information if they feel the doctor is listening. Good listening aids empathy (putting yourself in the patient's shoes). *Active listening* is demonstrated by the use of eye contact, posturing (e.g. head nodding) and responding or asking directly after the patients last response. For the interview to be purposeful, it is important that you encourage the patient to remain relevant to the purpose of the interview and redirect them if they go off at a tangent. If there is any doubt about a response it is OK to ask the patient for clarification. Sometimes, patients find it difficult to articulate their true problems and concerns, and both verbal and nonverbal cues help to shed more light on the underlying problem. An example of a *verbal cue* is a patient who has presented with heartburn and during the course of the consultation may say, 'my mother suffered with heartburn and turned out to have stomach cancer'. This patient may not be particularly bothered about the heartburn and instead be seeking reassurance that they do not have cancer. The good doctor can glean much information from a patient's gait, posture and general body language – so-called *nonverbal cues*. For example, excessive eye contact may suggest anger and aggression, whereas lack of eye contact can imply embarrassment and depression. Appropriate *touch* (handshake, putting arm around a distressed person) is also a powerful means of communication, building rapport and showing empathy. No doubt some people find it easier to use touch than others. As a general rule, avoid excessive touching, particularly if you are someone who is not comfortable with touching other people.

Giving information to patients: a protocol

To give information effectively to the patient it is important that you understand the information being given and convey it using language the patient will be able to understand. The following scheme can be used to give information to patients.

1   Know in your own mind what information you plan to give before the interview commences.
2   At the start of the interview summarise the patient's problems to date and find out their understanding of their condition.
3   Outline the structure of the interview.
4   Give information using appropriate language and even drawings if necessary. Try to be as specific as possible, avoiding vague terms and medical jargon. It is crucial that important information is given first, as evidence shows that patients are more likely to recall this following the inter-

view. It is OK to say that you will give an information leaflet following the interview and if appropriate they can be followed up by a specialist nurse.

5 Explore the patient's views about the information they have just received and encourage them to ask any questions they may have.

6 Conclude the interview by checking their understanding and, if appropriate, further management plan.

Giving lifestyle advice

It is becoming increasingly clear that for many conditions, disease prevention is better than cure. Hence doctors are often asked to give lifestyle advice and not surprisingly such cases often feature in station 4 (Communication skills and ethics). Common scenarios where lifestyle advice may be given include smokers, excessive alcohol consumption, obesity, unsafe sex, etc. Shown here is one possible scheme to give lifestyle advice taking the example of the smoker.

1 Ask the patient about their attitudes to their health. It is important to get an idea of whether the patient is pursuing a particular lifestyle that is detrimental to their health through choice or ignorance. The 'three S' health belief model can be used to explore further. How does the patient perceive their *susceptibility* to illness because of their lifestyle? For instance, a patient who has lost a close relative though lung cancer may be more concerned about their own habit and may be receptive to the idea of change. On the other hand, if the relatives survived to an old age despite smoking, the patient will consider his own habit to be of low risk. The perceived *seriousness* of the potential risk of their lifestyle also has implications on whether the patient wants to modify their lifestyle. For instance, the smoker may think of developing emphysema as an acceptable risk, but lung cancer as much more serious. The final S stands for *solutions*. This refers to the perceived benefit of changing their lifestyle. If we continue with the same analogy the smoker may realise that by

stopping cigarette smoking, their risk of lung cancer would dramatically reduce. Hence, the smoker would choose to make a lifestyle change because of the perceived benefit.

2 Once you have an idea about how the patient feels about their lifestyle and whether they can be motivated to make a change, you can then move on to giving the patient relevant information. It is crucial to keep the information specific and concise, without using medical jargon.

3 The third stage is to negotiate a plan to make the lifestyle change. Most people find lifestyle difficult to initiate and even harder to maintain. Realistic and achievable targets need to be discussed.

4 You should conclude the interview by giving the patient a long-term support mechanism such as a contact with a support group. Studies show that written information is both desired by patients and effective, particularly when used as an adjunct to verbal information. Hence, you can offer to supply the patient with written information in the form of a pamphlet or booklet.

References

Backer B, Hannon R and Russell N (1994) *Death and Dying: understanding and care* (2e). Delmar Publications, Albany, NY.

British Medical Association, the Resuscitation Council (UK) and the Royal College of Nursing (2001) Decisions relating to cardiopulmonary resuscitation. *J Med Ethics.* 27: 310–16.

Faden R and Beauchamp TL (1986) *A History and Theory of Informed Consent.* Oxford University Press, Oxford, and New York, NY.

Kübler-Ross E (1969) *On Death and Dying.* Tavistock Publications, London.

Maguire P, Fairbairn S and Fletcher C (1989) Consultation skills of young doctors: benefit of undergraduate feedback training in interviewing. In: M Stewart and D Roter (eds) *Communicating with Medical Patients.* Sage Publications, Thousand Oaks, CA, USA.

Quill TE, Dresser R and Brock DW (1997) The rule of double effect – A critique of its role in end-of-life decision making. *N Eng J Med.* 337: 1768–71.

Chapter 2

The cases

Guidelines issued by the Royal College of Physicians (RCP) for host centres when writing scenarios for station 4 (Communication skills and ethics) are as follows:

1 The scenario should relate to everyday clinical practice and must not be too obscure and complex. It should not rely on detailed medical knowledge of any one condition, investigation, current management or prognosis.
2 The scenario should clearly define the task involved and what is expected of the candidate, e.g. obtaining consent for a procedure or discussing proposed management following diagnosis.
3 The scenario should be such as to sustain a 14-minute discussion between the candidate and the surrogate/patient.
4 The scenario should not be so complex that the surrogate/patient cannot play the role required.
5 The topic should, wherever possible, be a universal problem applicable to global medicine. It must not be such that the candidate needs detailed knowledge of UK law.
6 It is desirable that the scenario should have an ethical component as it is difficult for examiners to sustain a five-minute discussion based on a scenario entirely confined to communication skills.
7 Patient organisations oppose the description of patients by their diagnoses, believing that this stigmatises them, e.g. referring to 'epileptics', 'diabetics' and 'acromegalics' is unacceptable. Patients should be referred to as patients with epilepsy, diabetes, acromegaly, etc.
8 Abbreviations should be avoided wherever possible. Universally accepted abbreviations such as ECG and CXR are

allowable, but abbreviations for investigations, e.g. PCR, or organisations, e.g. DVLA, etc., may differ between countries and are therefore not allowable.

9 Emotionally charged topics need not be avoided provided the surrogate is well trained and experienced in role-playing. However, topics that involve particularly sensitive issues, e.g. sexual history, are best avoided.

It is worth taking a little time to study these guidelines. In particular it should be noted that the case must be a common clinical scenario and not obscure and complex, and there should be a well-defined task for the candidate. While some appreciation of law is required, you are not expected to have the knowledge of a lawyer.

While there are many possible cases it is perhaps useful to know that in broad terms the sorts of case you are likely to get in this section can be subdivided into four categories, which include:

- breaking bad news
- counselling patients
- discussion with relatives
- discussion with colleagues.

The following cases are broadly presented under these headings. However, it must be appreciated that this classification is arbitrary and there is often overlap between these broad categories. For instance, you may be asked to break bad news to a relative.

Breaking bad news

'When in doubt, tell the truth'
(Mark Twain)

Bad news is any information that alters a patient's perspective of the future in a negative way. It can come in many forms, such as the diagnosis of a serious condition such as cancer or a chronic illness like diabetes mellitus, or informing relatives about the illness in or the loss of a loved one. Withholding bad news from patients was commonly practised until recently. A survey conducted in 1961 (Oken, 1961) revealed that 88 per cent of doctors routinely withheld cancer diagnoses, and when they did disclose the diagnosis, it was often through euphemisms such as 'growth'. However, the same study and others since have shown that most patients wish to be informed of their diagnosis, which allows them to make informed choices. Hence, in recent years the paternalistic model of patient care has been replaced by an emphasis on disclosure and patient autonomy.

Breaking bad news is not something that most doctors enjoy and there are numerous stories about how unskilled physicians blundered their way through an important conversation, sometimes resulting in harm to the patient. I remember well when I was a medical student on an attachment with a breast surgeon who, during the course of his ward rounds, after a few friendly preliminaries would then say something like, '. . . well, we've got the results back and I'm sorry love but you've got cancer'. This was followed by a supposedly kind smile and sometimes a pat on the shoulder before moving on to the next patient. Some physicians contend that breaking bad news is an innate skill – like perfect pitch – that cannot be acquired otherwise. This is incorrect and it is certainly something that can be acquired with practice. Physicians who are good at discussing bad news with their patients usually report that breaking bad news is a skill that they have worked hard to learn. Furthermore, studies of physician education demonstrate that communication skills can be learned, and have effects that persist long after the training is finished.

The most important factors for patients when they receive bad news are the physician's competence, honesty and the use of straightforward language.

A protocol for breaking bad news

There is no straightforward way of breaking bad news and it is something that needs to be adapted to the individual patient and the news to be given to them. The following is a suggested strategy for case scenarios where you have to break bad news. It is based on Robert Buckman's six-step protocol for breaking bad news (Buckman, 1994; Maguire and Faulkner, 1988).

1 Getting started

Once the consultation has started, do your best to ignore the examiners. Ideally, manoeuvre the chairs so that your back is to them, without making it obvious to them as they may take offence! Do your best to imagine that you are in the clinic for real. Greet the patient enthusiastically, without being over-familiar. You may want to ask them if there is someone else who has come with them to the clinic. There never is of course, but it shows that you are thinking. It is best to imagine that this is a real patient in a real setting. Avoid the temptation of getting straight to the business of breaking the bad news. Instead try to establish rapport and get some background information. This has to be tailored to each patient and scenario, and the patient will to some extent dictate it. For instance, they may appear very impatient and demand to know the results from their investigations. It would thus be inappropriate for you to 'beat about the bush' and move on to stage two. In most cases, the patient will be more compliant and willing to listen. Often, it is a good idea to get some insight into the patient's social set-up and support networks, for example who they live with, etc. By this time you should have established some sort of rapport with the patient.

2 Set the agenda

Establish the reason why the two of you are here having this discussion.

3 Finding out how much the patient knows or suspects

By asking a question such as, 'What have you already been told about your illness?' you can begin to understand what the patient has already been told ('I have lung cancer, and I need surgery'), or how much the patient understood about what's been said ('the doctor said something about a spot on my chest X-ray'), the patient's level of technical sophistication ('I've got a T2N0 adenocarcinoma'), and the patient's emotional state ('I've been so worried I might have cancer that I haven't slept for a week').

4 Fire a 'warning shot'

You may have the opportunity to hint that you are about to break bad news, but avoid clichés such as, 'I'm afraid the news is bad . . .'.

5 Breaking the news

Keep it clear. The temptation is to rush into the diagnosis, but it is best to break the news at the patient's pace and in manageable chunks, and be sure to stop between each chunk to ask the patient if they understand ('I'm going to stop for a minute to see if you have any questions'). Long lectures are overwhelming and confusing. Remember to translate medical terms into English, and don't try to teach pathophysiology. For the more aware patient (this is the likely scenario for the exam) you may simply need to tell them the news.

6 The golden silence

Pause to let the news sink in.

7 Responding to the patient's feelings

If you don't understand the patient's reaction, you will leave a lot of unfinished business, and you will miss an opportunity to be seen as a caring physician. Learning to identify and acknowledge a patient's reaction is something that definitely improves with experience if you're attentive, but you can also simply ask ('Could you tell me a bit about what you are feeling?').

8 Planning and follow-through

At this point you need to synthesise the patient's concerns and the medical issues into a concrete plan that can be carried out in the patient's system of healthcare. Outline a step-by-step plan, explain it to the patient, and contract about the next step. Be explicit about your next contact with the patient ('I'll see you in clinic in two weeks'), or the fact that you won't see the patient ('I'm going to be rotating off service, so you will see Dr Smith in clinic'). Give the patient a phone number or a way to contact the relevant medical caregiver if something arises before the next planned contact.

What if the patient starts to cry while I am talking?

You must remember that the patient used in the exam may well be a professional actor who takes their role very seriously. In general, it is better simply to wait for the person to stop crying. If it seems appropriate, you can acknowledge it ('Let's just take a break now until you're ready to start again'), but do not assume you know the reason for the tears (you may want to explore the reasons now or later). Most patients are somewhat embarrassed if they begin to cry and will not continue for long. It is nice to offer a tissue if they are readily available (something to plan ahead), but try not to act as if tears are an emergency that must be stopped, and don't run out of the room; you want to show that you're willing to deal with anything that comes up.

References

Buckman R (1994) *How to Break Bad News: a guide for health care professionals.* Papermac, London.

Maguire P and Faulkner A (1988) Improve the counselling skills of doctors and nurses in cancer care. *BMJ.* **297**: 847–9.

Oken D (1961) What to tell cancer patients: a study of medical attitudes. *JAMA.* **175**: 1120–8.

Case 1: Pancreatic cancer with poor prognosis

Candidate information

You are the SHO in a gastroenterology clinic.

Please read the scenario below. You may make notes on the paper provided. When the bell sounds enter the examination room to begin the consultation.

Patient: Mr James Cummings

Age: 67 years

You are about to see the last patient in the clinic. Normally, a consultant supervises you, but she has had to leave early to attend an academic meeting. This patient was initially referred to the gastroenterology clinic with jaundice and abnormal liver biochemistry. At the last visit an abdominal mass could be palpated and a CT scan was requested. The CT scan has shown a bulky mass in the head of the pancreas with vascular encasement. There are also enlarged lymph nodes in the coeliac trunk. The report suggests that this is likely to represent an inoperable pancreatic cancer, and further evaluation with ERCP is advised. If appropriate, a stent can be placed. Your objective is to relay this information to Mr Cummings.

You have 14 minutes to communicate with the patient followed by one minute for reflection before discussion with the examiners. You are not required to examine the patient.

Patient information

Mr James Cummings

Aged 67 years

This man was referred to the gastroenterology clinic suffering with weight loss, lassitude and jaundice. During the clinic visit the doctor thought that she could feel a mass in the abdomen. At that visit the doctor did mention the possibility of this turning out to be something serious and thought the best way forward was to investigate further with a CT scan, which has since been carried out. The radiographer who carried out the CT scan did not comment on the findings, but did look somewhat concerned about the result. At the appointment today the patient expects to find out the results of the CT scan and a comprehensive plan for future management. The patient is extremely concerned that this may turn out to be a cancerous growth, but is optimistic that if it does turn out to be cancer it can be readily treated.

Possible prompts

- Can it be cured?
- I used to drink heavily – could that have caused it?
- What treatments are available?
- What does this ERCP involve?
- How long have I got to live?
- I'm constantly feeling nauseous – will that get worse?
- Will I experience a lot of pain?
- Will I need to stay in hospital towards the end?

Possible interview plan

- Greet the patient and introduce yourself to him.
- Set the agenda. Confirm that he had been seen by the consultant in her clinic and she had organised a scan and he is here to discuss the findings.
- Ask about his understanding of his illness and the tests carried out thus far. If he is completely off the mark, some groundwork needs to be done before the bad news can be broken. Alternatively, if he has a good comprehension of

the tests done to date, it may be easier to break the bad news.

- 'Fire the warning shot.' An appropriate remark may be, 'Well, we've received the report from your recent CT scan and it does show an abnormality.'
- Break the bad news, explaining to the patient that the scan has shown a cancer in the pancreatic gland and that this is not likely to be curable.
- Pause and let the news sink in (the golden silence).
- Respond to the patient's feelings in an empathetic manner. Answer any immediate questions that he may have.
- Plan the follow-through and the need to carry out an ERCP examination, which will be organised at the next available list. If you do not feel confident in explaining the procedure (specialist knowledge is not required here), simply say that you will provide him with a detailed leaflet or alternatively give him the opportunity to speak with one of the endoscopists beforehand. Remember, in the hypothetical world of the PACES exam, you always have access to leaflets, to specialist nurses and can make an appointment for the patient to see just about anybody!

Ethical issues and other discussion points

The candidate should be asked to identify the ethical issues raised in this case and how they would address them. The framework for discussion should include consideration of the underlying ethical principles, in particular the *autonomy* of the patient and their right to be involved in the decision-making process. Contrast this with the 'old-fashioned' paternalistic model of patient care, where bad news was kept from the patient.

The candidate should be able to deliver the bad news in a clear and concise manner without too much stalling and avoidance of the discussion.

Candidates should understand that patients react in different ways to bad news. But generally speaking they experience various stages suggested by Kübler-Ross (*see* p. 15). These stages include denial, anger, bargaining, depression and finally acceptance of the bad news.

Case 2: The young patient diagnosed with malignant melanoma

Candidate information

You are the SHO in a dermatology clinic.

Please read the scenario below. You may make notes on the paper provided. When the bell sounds enter the examination room to begin the consultation.

Patient: Miss Simone Dudley

Age: 24 years

This 24-year-old holiday rep had been referred urgently to the clinic with a lesion on her thigh, suspiciously like a malignant melanoma. A biopsy taken at her first visit has confirmed a melanoma. Also, the patient had been complaining of lethargy, abdominal pain and distension, and a recent ultrasound scan of the abdomen is strongly suggestive of multiple metastases. The biopsy and the scan were reviewed at the weekly dermatology department meeting and it is felt that the patient has advanced melanoma that cannot be cured. Your objective is to explain the diagnosis and answer any questions she may have.

You have 14 minutes to communicate with the patient followed by one minute for reflection before discussion with the examiners. You are not required to examine the patient.

Patient information

Miss Simone Dudley

Aged 24 years

This holiday rep has spent the last five years working in Greece. Prior to this illness she enjoyed excellent health, was a non-smoker and drank 20 units of alcohol each week. Some months ago, she noticed a dark, itchy lesion on her left thigh and saw a local doctor in Greece, who felt it was probably just an insect bite and reassured her. However, over the next two months she progressively deteriorated with lethargy, abdominal pain and distension, and the lesion grew larger and more pigmented. Hence she decided to leave her job and come back to the UK for further tests. Her GP was concerned about the lesion on her leg and organised a prompt review in the dermatology clinic as well as an abdominal ultrasound scan to investigate the distension and pain. At her first visit to the dermatology clinic a biopsy had been taken and the doctor had commented that there was a possibility that the lesion could turn out to be cancerous. Today she has returned to the clinic to get the result of the biopsy and the ultrasound scan, which she had in the interim. She is keen for her health problems to be cured, enabling her to return to her job in Greece. If she takes much more time off work, she runs the risk of losing her job. However, she is extremely anxious about the possibility of cancer and when the doctor confirms that it is cancer, it will come as devastating news that she will find very difficult to accept.

Possible prompts

- When can I go back to work?
- Is it serious and can it be cured?
- Will I need an operation?
- Oh my God – you mean it can't be cured?
- What about my job? What shall I tell them?
- How long have I got to live?

Possible interview plan

- Greet the patient and introduce yourself to her.
- Set the agenda. Confirm her previous attendance to the clinic when a biopsy was taken and that she has returned to discuss the findings.
- Ask about her understanding of the investigations carried out to date and what her expectations are.

- 'Fire the warning shot.' One suggestion is, 'The results of the biopsy are back and it does show an abnormality.'
- Break the bad news. Say that the biopsy findings show a cancer. It is crucial that you are unambiguous. If you feel that the patient would understand the significance of malignant melanoma, then this term may be preferable to cancer as it is more accurate. However, some patients may be falsely reassured that they do not have a cancer.
- Pause and let the news sink in (the golden silence).
- Respond to the patient's feelings in an empathetic manner. Answer any immediate questions that she may have.
- Go on to explain the advanced nature of the disease inasmuch as that it has spread to the liver and cannot be treated. Some people may feel that this bit of the news – i.e. the incurable nature of the condition – is more devastating than being told that she has a cancer. Hence you must again pause and let this bit of information sink in and respond to any immediate concerns. It can be appreciated that in a finite amount of time (14 minutes) only a limited amount of information can be given. It is best not to feel pressurised and feel that you have to get everything in. They will give credence to the manner in which information is given to the patient and be less concerned about the amount of information.
- Plan the follow-through: contact details for a nurse specialist who can be contacted as the patient requires more information.

Discussion
Similar issues as apply to case 1.

Case 3: Hodgkin's lymphoma

Candidate information

You are the SHO working on an infectious diseases ward.

Please read the scenario below. You may make notes on the paper provided. When the bell sounds enter the examination room to begin the consultation.

Patient: Mr Nilesh Patel

Age: 31 years

This Indian man was admitted to hospital with lethargy, weight loss and night sweats. He has been living in the UK for nine months and is studying for a masters degree in engineering (MEng). Clinical examination had shown cervical lymph node enlargement, which had been biopsied. Upon admission, there was a high clinical suspicion of tuberculosis and he had been started on treatment empirically. However, his lymph node biopsy has come back showing Hodgkin's lymphoma, which had not been previously suggested. You need to explain the revised diagnosis, and how his management is likely to alter. You must also answer any questions that he may have.

You have 14 minutes to communicate with the patient followed by one minute for reflection before discussion with the examiners. You are not required to examine the patient.

Patient information

Mr Nilesh Patel

Aged 31 years

This 31-year-old Indian man has been living in the UK for approximately nine months. He is currently studying for a masters degree in engineering (MEng). He was admitted to hospital with lethargy, weight loss and night sweats. In hospital, the doctors felt that he probably has tuberculosis and treatment was started. There was a swelling in the neck, which the medical team decided to investigate with a biopsy, and the doctor has now arranged to have a discussion with Mr Patel with the biopsy results. Mr Patel is very keen to leave hospital and get back to his studies, which are being financed by loans taken out by his family. Tuberculosis carries some stigma in his own community and he is keen that he is treated confidentially. When the doctor gives him the news that they have found a cancer on the biopsy, Mr Patel will be initially surprised and think that they have made a mistake, as his diagnosis is TB. However, it will be devastating when it sinks in that he has cancer.

Possible prompts

- Have you come to tell me I have TB?
- I must please ask you to keep my information confidential. I don't want people to find out that I have TB.
- When can I leave the hospital and get back to my studies?
- This is costing my family a lot of money and I don't want to stay in hospital unnecessarily.
- I don't understand; the other doctors told me I had TB.
- Lymphoma? I've never heard of this condition – is it serious?
- Am I going to die? How long have I got to live?
- Can you cure it then?

Possible interview plan

- Greet the patient and introduce yourself to him.
- Set the agenda by saying that you have come to discuss the biopsy finding with him.
- Ask about his understanding of the investigations carried out to date and what his expectations are. He may say that he expects it to confirm TB, in which case you must elaborate and explain to him that there are other conditions that can give an identical clinical picture. Go on to explain that this can include a form of cancer known as lymphoma.

This is the warning shot. He will not be expecting to be told that he has cancer. But at least now the notion will be there.

- Break the bad news. Say that the biopsy findings show that he has lymphoma, which is a type of cancer.
- Pause and let the news sink in (the golden silence).
- Respond to the patient's responses in an empathetic manner. Answer any immediate questions that he may have.
- Go on to explain the nature of the disease and its implications. It is perhaps appropriate to be optimistic with this case and emphasise that there are potentially curative treatments available. But specialists will need to be involved and the disease has to be staged before treatment is initiated.
- Plan the follow-through. Say that you will organise an urgent review by one of the haematologists, who may take over the patient's care and organise further management strategies.

Discussion

Similar issues as apply to case 1.

Case 4: Multiple sclerosis

Candidate information

You are the SHO in a neurology clinic.

Please read the scenario below. You may make notes on the paper provided. When the bell sounds enter the examination room to begin the consultation.

Patient: Mrs Amanda Wilcox

Age: 32 years

This lady has phoned up and brought her clinic appointment forward to discuss the results from recent investigations. She was initially referred by her GP with blurred vision. The clinical history was suggestive of multiple sclerosis. Subsequent investigations included a lumber puncture and an MRI scan. Results from both investigations are back now and are strongly suggestive of multiple sclerosis. Your objective is to explain the likely diagnosis and what implications this has for her.

You have 14 minutes to communicate with the patient followed by one minute for reflection before discussion with the examiners. You are not required to examine the patient.

Patient information

Mrs Amanda Wilcox

Aged 32 years

This lady developed blurred vision in one eye some months ago and was referred to a neurologist. She was seen by the consultant, who mentioned the possibility of multiple sclerosis (MS), although said it was probably unlikely and organised further tests, which have now been carried out. Since the hospital appointment, Mrs Wilcox has been extremely anxious about this turning out to be MS, especially as she 'read up' on the condition using the Internet. She was due to come back to the clinic in two weeks' time, but because of her anxiety she has brought the appointment forward. She normally works as a librarian and lives with her husband and three children, the youngest of whom is two years old. She is concerned that if she does turn out to have multiple sclerosis, she will lose her job and end up incapacitated and in a wheelchair. She is particularly concerned about the welfare of her children and her husband not being able to cope with her illness.

Possible prompts

- Am I likely to end up in a wheelchair?
- Am I likely to die from this?
- Will I go blind?
- But I feel absolutely fine now . . .
- Is there a cure for this?
- Are my children at risk?

Possible interview plan

- Greet the patient and introduce yourself to her.
- Set the agenda. Confirm with her that she has brought her appointment forward to discuss the results of the investigations organised at the previous clinic visit.
- Ask about her understanding of why the investigations were carried out and what had been discussed with her at the last visit.
- 'Fire the warning shot.' One suggestion is, 'The MRI scan has been reported and does suggest a problem.'
- Break the bad news. Explain that both the MRI scan and the lumbar puncture are strongly suggestive of multiple sclerosis.
- Pause and let the news sink in (the golden silence).
- Respond to the patient's feelings in an empathetic manner. Answer any immediate questions that she may have.
- Go on to discuss the details without giving her more information than she can handle. Remember, this is a

chronic condition, and there will be ample opportunity to discuss in the future. Be honest, but also try to reassure the patient. Emphasise that it is difficult to predict the course of the illness. Some people do deteriorate and end up in a wheelchair, but others can have a normal and productive life with only intermittent attacks.

- Plan the follow-through: contact details for a nurse specialist who can be contacted as the patient requires more information. It is worth telling her about self-help groups such as the MS Society.

Discussion and ethical issues

Generally similar issues to case 1. However, as this is a chronic illness where the patient is alive for many years and may gradually deteriorate, it is important that issues such as *living wills* (*see* p. 5) are also brought into the discussion.

Case 5: Mesothelioma

Candidate information

You are an SHO in a chest clinic.

Please read the scenario below. You may make notes on the paper provided. When the bell sounds enter the examination room to begin the consultation.

Patient: Mr Fred Fogarty

Age: 72 years

This gentleman was referred to the chest clinic with weight loss, shortness of breath and a grossly abnormal chest X-ray. Clinical history taken at his first visit showed that he had worked as a shipbuilder and had been exposed to asbestos. He had also smoked 20 cigarettes a day since the age of 16 years. Following the assessment it was felt that his X-ray and clinical history were consistent with a pulmonary malignancy, associated with asbestosis. A subsequent pleural biopsy has confirmed the diagnosis of a malignant mesothelioma. Your objective today is to explain to him that he has a noncurative malignancy, probably secondary to his previous exposure to asbestos.

You have 14 minutes to communicate with the patient followed by one minute for reflection, before discussion with the examiners. You are not required to examine the patient.

Patient information

Mr Fred Fogarty

Aged 72 years

Mr Fogarty was referred to the chest clinic with shortness of breath and weight loss. It was noted that he had an abnormal chest X-ray and the doctor who saw him initially had suggested that there was a possibility of cancer and that he should be investigated further with a CT scan and a pleural biopsy. As a young man, Mr Fogarty had worked as a shipbuilder and knows that he had been exposed to asbestos. He had also smoked approximately 20 cigarettes a day since the age of 16 years. Today he has returned to the clinic to get the results of his biopsy and is anxious about the possibility of cancer. In particular, Mr Fogarty is concerned about his wife, Edith. She suffers with acute anxiety attacks and he has looked after her over the years. If it turns out to be cancer, he feels that she will take the news badly. At his last visit the doctor had given him a leaflet highlighting the potential lung diseases that can be caused by asbestos. It had also mentioned that patients might be able to claim compensation and he is keen to explore this possibility.

Possible prompts

- Have you got the results of my test?
- Does it show anything to worry about?
- I've heard this term mesothelioma, but I don't understand it. Is it serious?
- I'm very worried about my wife, Edith; I don't know how she will take this news. I suspect she will be devastated.
- How will we manage? In your leaflet, it mentioned the possibility of making a claim. Can you tell me more?

Possible interview plan

- Greet the patient and introduce yourself to him.
- Set the agenda. Confirm the patient had previously been seen in the clinic and tests including a pleural biopsy had been organised. Go on to say that you hope to discuss the results of the biopsy with him today.
- Ask about his understanding of the investigations carried out and what his expectations are.
- 'Fire the warning shot.' One suggestion is, 'The biopsy result is back and it does show a problem.'
- Break the bad news. Explain that the biopsy result shows a cancer, which was probably caused by his previous exposure to asbestos.

- Pause and let the news sink in (the golden silence).
- Respond to the patient's feelings in an empathetic manner. Answer any immediate questions that he may have.
- Go on to explain that the disease is not curable and you can only offer supportive and symptomatic treatments. If he specifically enquires about his prognosis, explain that generally people do not live more than two years from the time of diagnosis, but it is difficult to predict the course of the disease in each individual.
- If he asks about claiming industrial benefits, explain that he is eligible to claim benefits and the medical team will assist in any way possible. Benefits must be claimed through his local Department for Work and Pensions office.
- Plan the follow-through. He should receive an appointment to be reviewed again in the clinic and should be given the contact details for a lung cancer nurse specialist, who can be contacted as the patient requires help or information.

Asbestos and lung disease

In the past asbestos was commonly used in the building trade. Now it is uncommon and carefully controlled. The fibres enter the lung by inhalation and cause fibrosis, which can progress to malignancy. White asbestos (chrysolite) is the least fibrogenic, while blue asbestos (crocidolite) is the most fibrogenic. Brown asbestos (amosite) is the least common and of intermediate fibrogenicity.

Industrial claims

Doctors need to be aware of the possibility of compensation where disease is thought to be secondary to occupation. Diseases to consider compensation for include:

- asbestos-related disease
- occupational asthma and other industrial lung diseases
- noise-induced hearing loss
- vibration white finger
- repetitive strain injury (e.g. tenosynovitis).

Case 6: HIV positive

Candidate information

You are the SHO in the infectious diseases clinic.

Please read the scenario below. You may make notes on the paper provided. When the bell sounds enter the examination room to begin the consultation.

Patient: Mr Jeffrey Vaughn

Age: 28 years

You are asked to see this homosexual man. He has returned unexpectedly at the end of the clinic to find out the result of his HIV test, which he had taken voluntarily the previous week. He is very keen to know the result, which has come back positive. Your job is to explain the result to him and how you will manage him. Also you need to ensure that his partner is not at risk of contracting the disease.

You have 14 minutes to communicate with the patient followed by one minute for reflection before discussion with the examiners. You are not required to examine the patient.

Patient information

Mr Jeffrey Vaughn

Aged 28 years

This man has been a practising, anoreceptive homosexual for over 10 years. He has had multiple sexual partners over the years and rarely asked his partners to use condoms. Now, he has been in a stable relationship for two years and decided to have his HIV status checked when he found out that one of his previous partners had developed AIDS. He is very concerned about the possibility of being HIV positive. He is also concerned about telling his partner, who is largely unaware of his previous promiscuity, and about losing his job as a chef, which is a passion for him.

Possible prompts

- Are you telling me I have AIDS?
- Can this be cured?
- Will my partner have the condition?
- Do I have to tell my employers?
- How do I tell my partner?

Possible interview plan

- Greet the patient and introduce yourself to him.
- Set the agenda. Confirm that the man has previously had an HIV test and has returned today to get the result.
- Enquire about his expectation. If he feels that it is likely to be positive, ask about why he feels this way and vice versa.
- 'Fire the warning shot.' One suggestion is, 'The HIV test result is back and it is of some concern.'
- Break the bad news. Tell him the result was positive.
- Pause and let the news sink in (the golden silence).
- Respond to the patient's feelings in an empathetic manner. Answer any immediate questions that he may have.
- Go on to discuss the implications the positive result has for him. Remember, issues such as job and insurance discrimination do not need to be covered here, as they should have been discussed at the pretest counselling session (*see* case 20).
- It is important to emphasise that being HIV positive is not the same as having AIDS.
- It is pertinent to advise him to practise safe sex to reduce the risk of infecting others. Moreover, he should disclose his HIV status to his present and (if possible) past partners with whom he has had unprotected sex, so that they can be tested.
- Plan the follow-through. He should get contact details for people who can continue to give him information, help and support. Tell him that you will give him a leaflet, which has

the contact details for the Terence Higgins Trust, which can offer individuals advice and self-help. Also give him details for a specialist nurse.
- Ask if he has any other questions and close the interview.

Discussion points

The candidate should introduce himself to the patient and establish a rapport with him. He should agree with him that they are here to discuss the patient's HIV test. The candidate should explore the patient's concerns in an empathetic and non-judgemental manner before telling the patient that he is HIV positive in a clear manner and ensure that he has understood. It is particularly important that the candidate clarifies that this is HIV and not AIDS, and ensures that the patient understands that this information is confidential, but if he fails to disclose it to insurers, etc., then the policy may be void. The candidate should be able to answer any questions that the patient may have and agree a future plan of action including information on help groups.

A particularly pertinent issue that relates to this case is that of confidentiality and third-party risk. Remember that confidentiality is the cornerstone of the doctor–patient relationship, and it supports the principle of patient autonomy, which emphasises the patient's right to control over his life. The doctor must respect and maintain this confidentiality unless there is a greater good, such as the risk to the partner of a patient when you know the patient refuses to practise safe sex.

Case 7: The Down's syndrome pregnancy

Candidate information

You are the SHO working on a medical ward.

Please read the scenario below. You may make notes on the paper provided. When the bell sounds enter the examination room to begin the consultation.

Patient: Mrs Lynn Russell

Age: 45 years

This lady is in hospital with rheumatoid arthritis and is currently being treated with steroids and seems to be improving. She is also in the first trimester of her pregnancy, which is being managed jointly with the obstetric team. Initial blood tests and her age put her into the high-risk category for her baby to have congenital defects. She went on to have an amniocentesis, which confirms Down's syndrome. The obstetrician has called you with the result and has asked you to inform her of this diagnosis and discuss the possibility of abortion with her.

You have 14 minutes to communicate with the patient followed by one minute for reflection before discussion with the examiners. You are not required to examine the patient.

Patient information

Mrs Lynn Russell

Aged 45 years

This lady was admitted to hospital with pain in her hands, thought to be secondary to a flare-up of rheumatoid arthritis. Now the disease seems to be settling with steroid and analgesic therapy. Prior to the admission, Mrs Russell had found out that she was pregnant. She has one seven-year-old girl and very much wants another child and was very happy to find out that she was pregnant. But the initial assessment had put the pregnancy at high risk for Down's syndrome and the obstetrician looking after her had recommended an amniocentesis. Mrs Russell is extremely anxious about the result. One of the doctors has asked to speak with her and she anticipates that this will be about the amniocentesis result. She will be very upset when she finds out that the baby has Down's syndrome. Whether or not to abort the pregnancy will be an incredibly difficult decision to make and one that she will almost certainly not be able to make at this meeting.

Possible prompts

- Was the test normal?
- How can you tell the baby has Down's syndrome just by analysing the fluid in the womb?
- Do I have to have an abortion? Can I choose not to?
- Has the baby got Down's syndrome because of the rheumatoid arthritis?
- Could my treatment have caused it?
- If I became pregnant again, will the baby have Down's syndrome?

Possible interview plan

- Greet the patient and introduce yourself to her.
- Set the agenda. Confirm that she has had an amniocentesis and is awaiting the result and try to establish a rapport with the patient.
- Ask about her expectations and follow any verbal cues.
- 'Fire the warning shot.' One suggestion is, 'The obstetrician looking after you has asked me to speak with you regarding the test as he is concerned about the result.'
- Break the bad news. Tell her that the result shows a chromosomal defect consistent with Down's syndrome.
- Pause and let the news sink in (the golden silence).
- Respond to the patient's feelings in an empathetic manner. Answer any immediate questions that she may have.

- Go on to discuss the implications of the result with her. In particular you must explore her views.
- Broach the subject of abortion of the foetus and listen carefully to her responses. Remember, your job is not to persuade the lady to have an abortion (some people may even consider it outside the remit of a physician role), but simply to help her to make an informed choice.
- Plan the follow-through. Tell her that you will organise for her to speak with a genetic counsellor and an obstetrician.
- Ask if she has any other questions and close the interview.

Legal issues – abortion

The Abortion Act 1967 dictates abortion laws in England, Scotland and Wales. The law basically allows abortion if two doctors agree that continuation of the pregnancy may result in serious physical or mental health problems for the mother or existing children. Or there is a substantial risk that if the child were born it would suffer from such physical or mental abnormalities as to be seriously handicapped (what constitutes a 'serious handicap' is not addressed in the legislation). The Human Fertilisation and Embryology Act 1990 amended the Abortion Act, in particular it removed pre-existing links with The Infant Life Preservation Act 1929, which had made it illegal to 'destroy the life of a child capable of being born alive' (which was assumed to be 28 weeks). Hence termination can be carried out at any gestational age, provided it is justified by medical reasoning.

According to The Abortion Act 1967, doctors can refuse to participate in abortions because of a conscientious objection, provided that, in an emergency, necessary treatment can be provided to a woman at risk of death.

The pro-abortion lobby base their argument on the basis that the overriding principle is the woman's right to choose what happens to her body. Whereas, the anti-abortionists base their case on numerous ethical, moral and religious issues, the most compelling of which is the notion of the sanctity of all human life. There are others who choose to 'sit on the fence' in this debate and argue that abortion is wrong except in compelling circumstances such as the diagnosis of serious disease in the foetus.

Genetic screening and 'the new eugenics'

The eugenics (Greek, means 'good genes') movement began at least 100 years ago and became a powerful social force as it tried to create 'better humans through better breeding' and even sterilisation of undesirables. Now, similar ethical and moral dilemmas are increasingly becoming part of modern medicine. This is because of the availability of prenatal testing, genetic screening and, in the future, genetic manipulation and cloning. In the search for the ideal 'Citizen', there is a concern that people will be discriminated against because of their bad genes. For instance, will employers and insurers base their contracts on the basis of an individual's genetic make-up? Perhaps we are already practising the eugenics mindset by trying to exclude patients with Down's syndrome from our society. After all, many of these individuals are unique, intelligent human beings who enjoy great happiness. Should we be testing for this condition and then aborting high-risk pregnancies? Others may argue that know-ledge empowers doctors and patients to make appropriate decisions.

Clearly this is a minefield of ethical dilemmas. There are very few right and wrong answers here. It is very important that you think through some of the issues and have opinions on the controversy and debate.

Case 8: Death of husband

Candidate information

You are a medical SHO on call for the coronary care unit (CCU).

Please read the scenario below. You may make notes on the paper provided. When the bell sounds enter the examination room to begin the consultation.

Subject: Mrs Janice Levin

Age: 59 years

Re: husband, Mr Ron Levin, aged 64 years

You are asked to speak to Mrs Levin by the sister on CCU. Her husband, Mr Ron Levin, was a 64-year-old man who was admitted to the CCU on the previous evening, following an acute myocardial infarct. Prior to this he had been fit and well, although was known to smoke and suffered with hypertension. Mr Levin had been thrombolysed, and had been treated appropriately and urgently. However, during the night he had developed further chest pains and had a cardiac arrest from which he could not be resuscitated, despite a prolonged resuscitation, and subsequently died. His wife was informed of the deterioration over the telephone, but is unaware of the death. Sister has asked you to inform Mrs Levin that her husband has died and answer any questions she may have.

You have 14 minutes to communicate with the patient followed by one minute for reflection before discussion with the examiners.

Patient information

Mrs Janice Levin

Aged 59 years

Re: husband, Mr Ron Levin, aged 64 years

This lady's husband (Mr Ron Levin) was admitted to the CCU the previous evening when he developed chest pain and was diagnosed with an acute myocardial infarct. He was treated quickly and seemed to make a good recovery, and was alert and pain-free when she left him. Prior to this admission, Mr Levin had been a fit man. During the course of the night, Mrs Levin received a call from the hospital. The nurse had told her that her husband 'had taken a turn for the worse' and suggested she should come in to see him. Mrs Levin is extremely concerned about her husband, but is optimistic that he will make a full recovery. On arrival at the CCU, a nurse greeted her and asked her to wait in the relatives' room where a doctor would give her an update on his condition, before she is allowed to see him. The doctor will explain to her that her husband had another heart attack during the night and died. Mrs Levin will be devastated by this news.

Possible prompts

- Can you tell me how my husband is please? They are not letting me see him.
- Is he going to be OK?
- The doctor yesterday said he was going to be OK. What went wrong?
- Could anything have been done to save him?
- Can I see him please?
- Will they need to do a postmortem?

Possible interview plan

- Greet the lady and introduce yourself.
- Set the agenda. Confirm that she has been called back to the hospital by the nurse to discuss her husband.
- Enquire about her expectations. Briefly go into what prompted his admission and how she feels he is progressing.

- 'Fire the warning shot.' One suggestion is, 'During the night your husband developed some more chest pain and possibly had another heart attack.'
- Break the bad news. Go on to explain that Mr Levin's heart stopped beating, possibly because of another heart attack, and despite the best efforts of the medical team he died.
- Pause and let the news sink in (the golden silence).
- Respond to the patient's feelings in an empathetic manner. Answer any immediate questions that she may have.
- Do not feel pressured to speak – a gentle and empathetic manner may be more effective than words.
- Ask if she has any other questions and close the interview.

Discussion

Do you feel that you or the sister could have informed this lady of her husband's death down the telephone?

It is always ill-advised to break bad news over the telephone for at least two reasons.

1 It is unkind, as you do not know if the recipient of the news has any support to hand and how they will cope with the news.
2 You cannot be sure with whom you are discussing the matter and it could result in a serious breach of confidentiality.

Case 9: The sick daughter

Candidate information

You are a medical SHO on call for the coronary care unit (CCU).

Please read the scenario below. You may make notes on the paper provided. When the bell sounds enter the examination room to begin the consultation.

Subject: Mrs Nancy Berry

Age: 48 years

Re: daughter, Miss Paula Berry, aged 18 years

Paula Berry is an 18-year-old student who was brought to hospital after a severe asthma attack. Despite aggressive treatment by the paramedics, she went on to have a cardiac arrest while in casualty. Cardiopulmonary resuscitation was rapidly commenced, but she had a prolonged arrest of 25 minutes before output was obtained. She now has an output and is being ventilated, but the team are extremely pessimistic about her prognosis. Her pupils do not respond to light and gag reflexes are absent. The anaesthetist on call has arranged a transfer for her to the ITU. They plan to monitor her for 24 hours and if there is no improvement to switch the ventilator off. Discussion with her GP over the telephone suggests that Miss Berry was previously well, with her asthma under good control, and has never previously required hospital admission.

Her mother has just arrived at the hospital and is unaware of her daughter's condition. One of the nurses has taken her to the relatives' room and has asked you to speak with her. Your task is to have a discussion with Mrs Berry to explain the situation.

You have 14 minutes to communicate with the patient followed by one minute for reflection before discussion with the examiners.

Subject information

Mrs Nancy Berry

Aged 48 years

Re: daughter, Miss Paula Berry, aged 18 years

This lady was alarmed to hear that her 18-year-old daughter had been admitted to hospital with an asthma attack and has now arrived there to see how she is. Paula is a healthy and happy young student who only suffers with mild asthma, which is usually well controlled with inhalers. She is one of four children, but is both the youngest and the only daughter, and has always been the baby of the family. Upon arrival at the hospital a nurse has taken Mrs Berry to the relatives' room to speak with a doctor before seeing her daughter. She will be shocked to hear that her daughter had a severe asthma attack, which caused her heart to stop, requiring cardiopulmonary resuscitation. The doctor will explain to her that Paula is now on a ventilator and perhaps the worse news is that she is likely to have sustained irreversible brain damage and may already be 'brain dead'.

Possible prompts

- How is my daughter? Can I see her please?
- What caused this? She was fine this morning.
- Oh my God! What do you mean – cardiac arrest? She is only 18 years old.
- When can she come off the ventilator?
- Irreversible brain damage? Does that mean she will never wake up?
- Can I see her now, please?

Possible interview plan

- Greet the lady and introduce yourself.
- Set the agenda. Confirm that she has come to hospital to see her daughter who was admitted earlier in the day.

- Enquire about her expectations. Try to gain insight into what Mrs Berry understands about her daughter's illness.
- 'Fire the warning shot.' One suggestion is, 'Your daughter had a severe asthma attack and was extremely sick when she arrived at hospital.'
- Break the bad news. Go on to explain that Paula Berry had a prolonged cardiac arrest, which is likely to have caused irreversible brain damage and she will probably never regain consciousness.
- Pause and let the news sink in (the golden silence).
- Respond to the mother's feelings in an empathetic manner. Answer any immediate questions that she may have.
- Explain to her that it is difficult to predict her daughter's progress and that the medical and nursing team will keep her informed of any developments.
- Inform her that she will be able to see her daughter immediately. Ask if she has any other questions and close the interview.

Counselling patients

One of our key roles in hospital medicine is the diagnosis and treatment of chronic conditions. To deliver the best possible care, it is important that the patients are appropriately educated about their conditions and hence there is a frequent need to communicate with the patient. Hence, not surprisingly, such cases have made their way into the PACES exam.

Here follows a few general points regarding such cases.

- Patients are often experts on their conditions and it often helps to get an idea of their understanding before embarking on a major counselling session.
- Chronic conditions can be thought of in terms of the impact they have on a patient's life and conversely the patient's lifestyle may have an impact on the disease.
- Remember, in the hypothetical world of the PACES exam, you will have access to almost unlimited resources, which include: specialist nurses, information leaflets, patient associations, etc.
- Don't be frightened of showing initiative, for example by drawing a diagram to illustrate the colon in explaining ulcerative colitis to a patient.

Case 10: Lifestyle advice for diabetes mellitus

Candidate information

You are the SHO in the diabetes clinic.

Please read the scenario below. You may make notes on the paper provided. When the bell sounds enter the examination room to begin the consultation.

Patient: Mr Raymond Royce

Age: 52 years

This gentleman was recently diagnosed with diabetes mellitus by his GP and started on metformin. He has presented to the diabetes clinic for the first time. The GP's letter suggests that he would like to know how diabetes is likely to affect his lifestyle. He is particularly concerned about losing his job as a bus driver. He is overweight, smokes 20 cigarettes a day and drinks about four pints of beer each evening. Please advise him accordingly.

You have 14 minutes to communicate with the patient followed by one minute for reflection before discussion with the examiners. You are not required to examine the patient.

Patient information

Mr Raymond Royce

Aged 52 years

This gentleman has recently been diagnosed with diabetes mellitus and is currently taking metformin. He is overweight and leads a very sedentary lifestyle, working as a bus driver and spending his evenings either in the pub or at home watching television. He smokes 20 cigarettes a day and on average drinks about four pints of beer each evening. He is married with three children, although only one still lives at home. Mr Royce is concerned about his diagnosis of diabetes and how it will affect his lifestyle. He is particularly concerned about any impact it may have on his vocation as a bus driver as he has heard of people losing their PSV licences because they were diagnosed with diabetes. This gentleman is also worried about his eyesight, which has significantly deteriorated recently. He has not got round to having his eyes tested and has not mentioned this to anyone previously.

Possible prompts

- Will I end up on injections? I hate needles.
- Will I have to give up my job?
- Does my employer need to know about this condition?
- My eyesight has deteriorated – is it likely to be related?
- Is it a serious condition?

Possible interview plan

- Greet the gentleman and introduce yourself.
- Set the agenda. Confirm that he has been referred to this clinic after recent diagnosis of diabetes mellitus.
- Enquire about his expectations. Try to gain insight into Mr Royce's understanding of diabetes and whether he expects to make lifestyle modifications because of the diagnosis. Remember the three Ss (*see* p. 25):
  - *susceptibility:* explore his perception and understanding of possible complications related to his diagnosis of diabetes and his lifestyle. It is important for him to understand that this is a chronic condition that has implications for the rest of his life. Of particular importance is the aim to reduce the risk of macrovasular (cerebrovascular disease, peripheral vascular disease and ischemic heart disease) as well as microvascular (neuropathy, retinopathy and nephropathy) complications

- *seriousness:* does he believe that poor control of diabetes and his lifestyle is likely to have serious consequences for him?
- *solutions:* does he perceive a benefit in changing his lifestyle and will he consider doing so.
- Give lifestyle advice and negotiate change:
  - *diet:* avoid excess sugar in the diet. Eat fresh fruit and vegetables. For more formal dietary advice refer him to a dietician
  - *exercise regularly and lose weight*
  - *stop smoking* (*see* case 14) and moderate *alcohol* intake.
- Advice regarding driving (see below).
- Long-term support and follow-up. Effective management will involve a multidisciplinary approach, which will include doctors (especially diabetologists and opthalmologists), specialist diabetes nurse, dietician, chiropodist, etc.
- Ask if he has any other questions and close the interview.

Diabetes and driving

For specific advice refer to the DVLA website. Patients are allowed to drive cars and motorbikes if the diabetes is diet-controlled or well controlled on medication. Of particular importance is that they do not have episodes of hypoglycaemia (<4 mmol/l). Patients can also hold a licence to drive a large goods vehicle (LGV) or to drive a passenger services vehicle (PSV) if the diabetes is treated by diet alone or tablets, provided they do not have visual problems. However, since April 1991, it has been illegal to issue a LGV or PSV licence if the patient is insulin-dependent. Moreover, patients who change their treatments and go onto insulin automatically lose their licences. Drivers also need to be aware that poor vision as a result of retinopathy may result in the loss of their driving privileges.

Case 11: New diagnosis: rheumatoid arthritis

Candidate information

You are an SHO working on a medical ward.

Please read the scenario below. You may make notes on the paper provided. When the bell sounds enter the examination room to begin the consultation.

Patient: Mrs Anita Hull

Age: 44 years

This lady was admitted to hospital with progressive shortness of breath, which is being investigated. She also complained of joint pains, which had been worsening over some time. The previous day she had been seen by a rheumatologist, who had confidently diagnosed rheumatoid arthritis and started her on anti-inflammatory medication. Mrs Hull is concerned about her diagnosis and the impact it is likely to have on her lifestyle. She has asked to speak to a doctor. Your objective is to speak to her and answer any questions that she may have.

You have 14 minutes to communicate with the patient followed by one minute for reflection before discussion with the examiners. You are not required to examine the patient.

Patient information

Mrs Anita Hull

Aged 44 years

This lady was admitted to hospital three days ago, by her GP, with progressive shortness of breath. A comprehensive history had been taken and Mrs Hull had mentioned that she had suffered with pain in her joints, particularly her hands, for some time, but had not sought any medical advice for this although she had been self-medicating with paracetamol tablets. The admitting team had organised a rheumatological review and a consultant had seen her yesterday. He had commented on the inflammation in her hands and explained that she has rheumatoid arthritis and had started her on some tablets. He had also said that the breathing problems may be related.

This lady has previously been fit and well, and indeed works as a swimming instructor. She is divorced and has one daughter, aged 13 years.

Mrs Hull's grandmother had suffered with rheumatoid arthritis and she is concerned that her hands may become deformed like her grandmother's. She is also worried about the side effects of the medication she is on, the impact it will have on her lifestyle and whether there is a chance that her daughter will get the condition.

Possible prompts

- Yesterday, the doctor told me that I had rheumatoid arthritis. What exactly does this mean?
- Will my hands become deformed like my grandmother's?
- The other doctor said that my breathing might be related to the arthritis. How can this be possible?
- I'm concerned about the side effects of the tablets I'm on. Are they safe?
- Will my daughter get arthritis?
- Can I lead a normal life?

Possible interview plan

- Greet the lady and introduce yourself.
- Set the agenda. Confirm that she has asked to speak with a doctor after recent diagnosis of rheumatoid arthritis.
- Enquire about her understanding of this diagnosis and the possible implications for her.
- Information given must be free of medical jargon and where possible specific. It should include the following:

- The disease causes inflammation in the joints (you may have to explain what you mean by joints). It is thought to be autoimmune, i.e. the body reacts against the joints. The condition can lead to deformity, but the progress in each patient is unpredictable. Often there are isolated attacks with long periods where the disease is inactive. It is important to emphasise that many patients can lead normal and healthy lives.
- It is not an inherited condition, but patients with an affected relative are more likely to get the condition. Hence the risk of her daughter developing the disease is small.
- There has to be a balancing act between rest and exercise. As a general rule contact sports are best avoided and patients should be encouraged to protect their joints. However, low-impact exercise (and swimming is probably the best) should be strongly encouraged.
- There are a number of medications used to treat arthritis, which include analgesics, disease-modifying drugs (e.g. sulphasalazine, methotrexate, azathioprine, etc.) and now biologicals (such as anti-TNF drugs). They all have side effects but you need not go into details.

- Explore the lady's views about the information she has received and encourage her to ask any questions she may have.
- Explain to her that she will be followed up by a rheumatologist.
- Thank her and close the interview.

Case 12: Man with TB

Candidate information

You are the SHO working on the infectious diseases ward.

Please read the scenario below. You may make notes on the paper provided. When the bell sounds enter the examination room to begin the consultation.

Patient: Mr Gurmail Singh

Age: 37 years

Mr Singh was initially admitted with weight loss and a productive cough, after a prolonged visit to India. The initial chest X-ray was found to be abnormal and he was put into a side room (which is causing him to become considerably frustrated) for barrier nursing, pending further investigation. A sputum sample has come back positive for alcohol and acid-fast bacilli. Explain the diagnosis of tuberculosis and what the treatment entails. You are not expected to take a history.

You have 14 minutes to communicate with the patient followed by one minute for reflection before discussion with the examiners. You are not required to examine the patient.

Patient information

Mr Gurmail Singh

Aged 37 years

This gentleman was admitted to hospital with a cough and weight loss following a six-month trip to India. He has been barrier nursed since admission, which was over a week ago and he is not sure why, except that it is to prevent the spread of infection. Mr Singh was born in India, but moved to the UK as a child. He was working as a motor mechanic until he lost his job eight months previously. He normally lives with his wife and children, aged 2 and 8 years. Mr Singh is becoming increasingly frustrated with being confined to a small room and is desperate to find out what's going on and whether it is something serious. He is also concerned about any risks it may pose to his family.

Possible prompts

- I'm really fed up of being in this room. I wish someone would tell me what is going on.
- What exactly is TB and why did I get it?
- Will I infect my family?
- Will I have to take the tablets for the rest of my life?
- Do these medicines have side effects?
- Will I be cured after taking these medicines?
- Will I be able to get back to my job?

Possible interview plan

- Greet the gentleman and introduce yourself.
- Set the agenda. Explain that you have come to speak with him regarding his hospital admission.
- Enquire about his understanding of the reason for this admission to hospital.
- If he has no comprehension of why he is in hospital and isolated, explain to him that the admitting team suspected tuberculosis, which is an infective illness, and hence he was isolated.
- Go on to inform him that the test results do indeed confirm that he has TB and that this will require treatment with antibiotics. Remember your remit here is to simply inform the man of his diagnosis and management strategies. Hence you need not go into details of his treatments and possible side effects. Also, depending on the context in which the news is given to the patient and his possible perceptions, you may have to give him the diagnosis in a manner similar to the breaking bad news scenarios previously discussed.

- Remind him that this is an infective illness and hence his close contacts, particularly his family, will also need to be screened for the illness and, if appropriate, treated. Moreover, he must continue to be isolated until his sputum does not contain the bacteria responsible for TB ('smear negative').
- Summarise the discussion and ask whether he has any final questions.
- Thank him and close the interview.

TB and public health ethics

Tuberculosis is the world's leading infectious killer and is responsible for approximately two million deaths per annum (Dye *et al.*, 1999). People at the greatest risk of developing the condition include the poor, substance abusers, those infected with HIV and prison populations. These people also have the least access to treatment. Efforts to control TB include complex ethical considerations involving public health ethics. Generally, medical ethics focuses on individual patients and the preservation of their autonomy and dignity. Public health ethics concentrates on the protection and promotion of health in communities. One key ethical issue is balancing the patient's rights and autonomy with the protection of the community. Treatments such as directly observed therapy (DOT), detention and mandatory treatment entail loss of patient's autonomy. But these can be justified on the basis that they prevent greater harm to the community at large.

There has been considerable interest in public health ethics in recent years. As a general rule, if there is a programme set up to protect the public and it violates an individual's rights, it must fulfil the following criteria. It must be necessary, effective proportionally and burdens from it must be minimised (Childress *et al.*, 2001).

References

Childress JF, Faden RR, Gaare RD, Gostin LO, Kahn J, Bonnie RJ, Kass NE, Mastroianni AC, Moreno JD and Nieburg P (2001) Public health ethics: mapping the terrain. *J Law Med Ethics*. **30**: 170–8.

Dye C, Scheele S, Dolin P, Pathania V and Raviglione MC (1999) Consensus statement. Global burden of tuberculosis: estimated incidence, prevalence, and mortality by country. WHO Global Surveillance and Monitoring Project. *JAMA*. **282**: 677–86; 278: 838–42.

Case 13: New diagnosis: coeliac disease

Candidate information

You are the SHO in a gastroenterology clinic.

Please read the scenario below. You may make notes on the paper provided. When the bell sounds enter the examination room to begin the consultation.

Patient: Mrs Jayne Watkins

Age: 36 years

This lady has been investigated for persistent diarrhoea and weight loss. She had positive endomysial and tissue transglutaminase antibodies and a subsequent duodenal biopsy confirmed a diagnosis of coeliac disease. You should discuss the diagnosis, its management and possible implications with her. You are not expected to take a history from her.

You have 14 minutes to communicate with the patient followed by one minute for reflection before discussion with the examiners. You are not required to examine the patient.

Patient information

Mrs Jayne Watkins

Aged 36 years

This lady has suffered with persistent diarrhoea and weight loss for about six months. She was subsequently referred to a gastroenterologist and was seen in the clinic by a consultant gastroenterologist, who organised blood and stool tests as well as an endoscopy. She has now returned to the clinic to find out the results of her investigations. She is very anxious about her illness and is hoping that the investigations will have clarified the diagnosis.

Possible prompts

- Will I ever get back to normal?
- Which foods are safe for me to eat?
- I've read that I could get cancer from this condition. Is this true?
- Will my children get coeliac disease? Is it inherited?
- I've noticed a very itchy rash on my knees. Is that related?

Possible interview plan

- Greet the lady and introduce yourself.
- Set the agenda. Confirm that she initially presented with diarrhoea and weight loss and has had a series of investigations to find out the cause of her problems.
- Enquire about any previous discussions with the medical team and whether she was aware of specific illnesses, particularly coeliac disease.
- Explain to her that the tests, including the duodenal biopsy, confirm a diagnosis of coeliac disease.
- You need to explain in simple terms what implications this has for her. She needs to avoid wheat, barley and rye, or any foods that contain these. Oats are debatable, because they are not thought to have a direct effect on the disease, but commercially available oats are often contaminated by the other wheat germs.
- Say that you will arrange for a dietician to see the patient and provide her with a list of safe foods. Emphasise that the dietary changes are likely to be lifelong. The risk of not adhering to a strict diet may result in relapses of the coeliac disease and the consequences, which include anaemia and osteomalacia/osteoporosis.
- Go on to explain that coeliac disease is associated with an itchy vesicular rash, particularly affecting the elbows and shins. This usually settles with the dietary control, but occasionally requires drug treatment.
- It may be worth mentioning the slightly increased risk of intestinal lymphoma, but reassure her that the risk of this is

extremely small and you have informed her because she may hear about it somewhere else and become alarmed.

- Reassure her that it is not an inherited condition, but patients often do have a genetic susceptibility, e.g. if of Irish origin.
- Tell her about the Coeliac Society.
- Summarise the discussion and let her know that you will organise a follow-up in the clinic.
- Thank her and close the interview.

Case 14: New diagnosis: asthma

Candidate information

You are the SHO on a respiratory ward.

Please read the scenario below. You may make notes on the paper provided. When the bell sounds enter the examination room to begin the consultation.

Patient: Mr Phillip Yates

Age: 27 years

The nurse looking after this man has asked you to speak to him at his request. He was admitted to hospital with difficulty in breathing, which was diagnosed as acute severe asthma. Treatment with steroids and nebuliser therapy caused a rapid recovery (ITU was not required). Previously, Mr Yates had been fit and well and regularly played football. His discharge medication consists of salbutamol and Flixotide inhalers as well as prednisolone 40mg once daily for one week. Mr Yates is concerned about the impact this will have on his lifestyle. He smokes 15 cigarettes a day, plays football at the weekends and works as a book-keeper. Your task is to discuss the impact that the diagnosis of asthma will have on his lifestyle.

You have 14 minutes to communicate with the patient followed by one minute for reflection before discussion with the examiners. You are not required to examine the patient.

Patient information

Mr Phillip Yates

Aged 27 years

This gentleman was admitted to hospital with shortness of breath and was diagnosed with acute severe asthma. This was

treated with nebulisers and steroid tablets and he made a good
recovery over the next few days. He is now on various inhalers
and a reducing course of oral steroids and is nearly ready for
discharge from hospital. Prior to this admission, this gentleman
was fit and well, playing football regularly. He has been a smoker
for 10 years and currently smokes 10 cigarettes a day. He is very
keen to give up and has tried to on a number of occasions, but
this has proved unsuccessful. It has been particularly difficult as
he works as a book-keeper and everybody smokes in the shop.
He is worried about the long-term damage to health by
continuing to smoke. He is also concerned about the diagnosis
of asthma and what implications this has for him, and the side
effects of the medication he has been started on, particularly
whether it is safe for him to continue to play football. He has
asked to speak to a doctor to discuss these issues further.

Possible prompts

- Why did I have this attack out of the blue?
- What side effects will I get with these steroid tablets? I've
  heard they are very bad for you.
- Could I have died as a result of this attack?
- Will I be OK with going back to work?
- Will I be OK to start exercising?
- Does smoking set off an asthma attack?

Possible interview plan

- Greet the gentleman and introduce yourself.
- Set the agenda. Confirm that he has asked to speak with a
  doctor and that he was admitted to hospital with shortness
  of breath and was diagnosed with asthma.
- Enquire about his understanding of asthma.
- If he has a good, sound understanding of the condition,
  then you can build on it and fill in any gaps. Alternatively,
  give a clear and concise explanation of the condition.
- It is important to emphasise that asthma is a chronic
  condition, which is well controlled in the majority of
  patients who lead normal and healthy lives. It is important

that 'flare-ups' are prevented by regularly using his steroid inhaler. Moreover, if there are obvious exacerbating factors such as dust, these must be avoided.

- Encourage exercise and a healthy lifestyle.
- Smoking advice (see below). Ask if he has ever considered stopping or indeed has tried stopping. If he has not thought about it, tell him it is very important that he tries to stop and that there is help available, both in terms of medical therapy and counselling.
- Summarise the discussion and ask him if he has any other questions.
- Thank him and close the interview.

Smoking cessation

A report by the Royal College of Physicians – Nicotine Addiction in Britain (February 2000) – has shown that many people continue to smoke, not through choice, but because of their addiction to nicotine. Surveys have shown that the majority of smokers wish to quit, but find it difficult because of their addiction and the resultant withdrawal symptoms. There is also a fear of weight gain, which occurs in 80 per cent of people when they quit cigarettes.

Smoking cessation aids

There are two proven pharmaceutical aids to stopping smoking:
1 *Nicotine replacement therapy.* This is designed to help the smoker to break the habit while providing a reduced dose of nicotine to overcome withdrawal symptoms such as craving and mood changes. It is available in various forms, which include chewing gum, skin patches, tablets, nasal spray and inhalers. Studies have shown that this form of therapy doubles the chances of a smoker successfully quitting the habit.
2 *Bupropion (Zyban).* This drug works by desensitising nicotine receptors within the brain and again doubles the chances of a smoker successfully quitting the habit. However, it is only available on prescription under medical

supervision because of possible side effects, the most serious of which is the risk of fitting. This risk is estimated to be less than 1 in 1000, but other less serious side effects such as insomnia, dry mouth and headaches are more common.

Other cessation methods tried by smokers include *acupuncture* and *hypnosis,* but there is little in the way of scientific evidence for their efficacy. *Herbal cigarettes* are not recommended as an aid to giving up smoking because they produce both tar and carbon monoxide, and reinforce the habit of smoking, which smokers need to overcome. *Clinics and self-help groups* can be extremely beneficial in helping people quit. Indeed, a review of smoking cessation products and services found that smokers are up to four times more likely to stop smoking by attending specialist smokers' clinics than by using willpower alone. Charitable organisations such as QUIT (Tel: 0800 002200) and Action against Smoking and Health (ASH) can be used to gain further support and get details of local self-help groups.

Case 15: Following a heart attack

Candidate information

You are an SHO working on the coronary care unit (CCU).

Please read the scenario below. You may make notes on the paper provided. When the bell sounds enter the examination room to begin the consultation.

Patient: Mr Frank Collins

Age: 52 years

You are asked to speak to a 52-year-old man who has been under your care following an acute myocardial infarct. He was treated promptly with thrombolysis and now, three days later, is making a very good recovery. He is concerned about changes that he needs to make to his lifestyle. He was previously known to be a diet-controlled diabetic, smoker of 30 cigarettes per day and worked as a long-distance lorry driver. Your task is to speak to him and recommend any lifestyle adjustments and answer any questions that he may have.

You have 14 minutes to communicate with the patient followed by one minute for reflection before discussion with the examiners. You are not required to examine the patient.

Patient information

Mr Frank Collins

Aged 52 years

This lorry driver was admitted to hospital with severe chest pain and was subsequently diagnosed with an acute coronary syndrome. He is known to suffer with diabetes, which is diet-controlled, although he generally avoids checking his blood sugars and knows that he eats badly. This includes frequent stops at cafés for 'greasy' meals and sugary snacks, washed down with pots of coffee. He drinks approximately 20 units of alcohol per week and smokes 30 cigarettes per day. He is married and lives with his wife of 28 years and four children. Mr Collins does not understand the term 'acute coronary syndrome' and has asked to speak to a doctor to clarify this and to understand what implications it has for him. He is particularly worried about any impact on him working as a lorry driver.

Possible prompts

- Can you explain what a coronary syndrome is please?
- Will I have another heart attack?
- Is it OK to start exercising?
- How soon can I get back to my regular activities?
- How often should I exercise?
- When can I go back to work?
- It's an embarrassing question doctor, but will sex be safe?

Possible interview plan

- Greet the gentleman and introduce yourself.
- Set the agenda. Confirm that he has asked to speak with you regarding his diagnosis.
- Enquire about his understanding of his diagnosis.
- If he has no insight into his diagnosis then you have to explain to him in simple lay terms that he has had a heart attack, which occurs when the blood vessels supplying the heart are occluded. Reassure him that he was treated effectively in good time and is expected to make a good recovery.
- Question him about his lifestyle and ask whether he is motivated to improve it. Remember the three Ss (*see* p. 25):
  - *susceptibility*: explore his perception and understanding of possible complications related to his lifestyle and the possibility of him having another myocardial infarct
  - *seriousness*: does he believe that his poor lifestyle is likely to have serious consequences for him?
  - *solutions*: does he perceive a benefit in changing his life tyle and will he consider doing so?

- Give lifestyle advice and negotiate change:
  - *diet*: eat a calorie-controlled diet low in fat (I'm sure you all know about good and bad fats!). Eat fruit and vegetables. For more formal dietary advice, say that you will refer him to a dietician
  - *medications*: explain that a number of medicines such as aspirin and a 'cholesterol-lowering drug' have been started to prevent further heart disease and he must not stop them even if he feels well in himself
  - *exercise regularly and lose weight*: this needs to be developed at a gradual pace and should be supervised by a specialist (e.g. a post-MI rehab nurse). Warn him that overexertion may put a strain on the heart muscle and lead to a further heart attack. Warning signs include chest pain, prolonged shortness of breath, dizziness, blotchy skin, nausea and vomiting. Remember, exercise includes sexual activity, which needs to be avoided in the first few weeks after a heart attack
  - *stop smoking* (see case 14) and *moderate alcohol intake.*
- Advice regarding *driving*. As a general rule there is a 4-week ban for group 1 licences and a 6-week ban for group 2 licences.
- Reassure him that his rehabilitation is a gradual process that will be supervised and assisted by the medical team. But remind him that he is ultimately responsible for his health and it is imperative that he makes lifestyle adjustments to avoid a further heart attack in the future.
- Ask if he has any other questions and if not close the interview.

Case 16: New diagnosis: epilepsy

Candidate information

You are an SHO in a neurology clinic.

Please read the scenario below. You may make notes on the paper provided. When the bell sounds enter the examination room to begin the consultation.

Patient: Miss Rosa Fletcher

Age: 29 years

This lady had presented to a hospital casualty department following two fits and was reviewed by the medical registrar. She diagnosed epilepsy and started the patient on sodium valproate and discharged her with an outpatient CT scan of the head and an EEG. A consultant neurologist has reviewed the case notes and the investigation results and feels that they are in keeping with a diagnosis of epilepsy. Miss Fletcher has now come to her first outpatient appointment. Your task is to explain the diagnosis with her and discuss the relevant issues.

You have 14 minutes to communicate with the patient followed by one minute for reflection before discussion with the examiners. You are not required to examine the patient.

Patient information

Miss Rosa Fletcher

Aged 26 years

This lady presented to casualty some months ago following two fits. She had had a similar, but less severe, episode previously, but had not sought medical advice. The doctor who had seen her in hospital had told her that she had had a fit and started some tablets (sodium valproate 200 mg twice daily). After a short period of observation she had been discharged from hospital with investigations organised as an outpatient. There had been no further fits and she has arrived at the clinic to get the results of her investigation. Normally, she lives with her long-term boyfriend in a recently purchased house. There are no plans to have children at present (and she is on an oral contraceptive), but in due course they would like to get married and have children. At the time of her diagnosis she had been asked about any medication she might be on and had said that she was not, as she didn't consider the contraceptive pill as medication. The doctor had also advised Rosa that she must inform the DVLA of her diagnosis, and that she would not be permitted to drive until she was deemed medically fit. She had chosen to ignore this advice as she drives for a living, transport-ing children to and from school. She also holds a part-time job as a steel press operator. As a matter of routine her employers (who operate the minibus she drives) insist on a health insurance form to be countersigned by a doctor every three years. Her own GP has refused to sign the form and she brought it to the hospital, planning to ask the consulting doctor to sign it during the course of the interview. The doctor will explain to Miss Fletcher that it is illegal for her to continue driving and that she is putting her own and others lives, at risk and she must explain this to the DVLA. Reluctantly she agrees to stop driving and to inform the DVLA.

Possible prompts

- The doctor in hospital said I had a fit. Is epilepsy the same?
- I plan to have children in the future. Will that affect my epilepsy?
- I can't stop working, especially as we've now got a mortgage.
- Will you please sign this form for me?
- Do I have to inform the DVLA? What happens if I don't?

Possible interview plan

- Greet the lady and introduce yourself.
- Set the agenda. Confirm that she previously presented to

hospital following a fit and this appointment and the investigations she has had were organised as a result of this.

- Enquire about any discussions she had with the doctors at the time of her presentation and what she feels may be the cause of her fit.

- Explain to her that her symptoms and investigations are suggestive of epilepsy. Ask her how much she knows about this condition.

- If she lacks insight into the condition, explain to her that epilepsy is a condition where there is altered electrical activity in the brain, which can cause fits. There is medication available to control fits, but it must be taken regularly, even when patients are fit-free. Emphasise to her that it is important that we prevent fits from occurring as they can cause irreversible brain damage and even death.

- Advice regarding driving. As a general rule, diagnosis of epilepsy leads to an automatic ban from driving. For Group 1 licences this is one year, for group 2, 10 years. The licence holder is legally obliged (Road Traffic Act 1988) to inform the DVLA of any medical condition (including epilepsy) that may impair their driving.

- Ask Miss Fletcher if she drives. She tells you that she does and transports children to and from school, and indeed shows you a health questionnaire form that is required by her employers, which she would like you to sign.

- Explain to her that you certainly cannot sign the form and that she needs to stop driving straight away and if she refuses, you will have no option but to inform the DVLA yourself. She is endangering not only her own life, but also the lives of others.

- Upon reflection, she reluctantly agrees to stop driving and inform the DVLA.

- Also tell her to avoid using heavy machinery. She will tell you that she operates a steel press. Iterate the point that if she has a fit while operating the press it could result in serious injury.

- Tell her that anti-epileptics (anticonvulsants) can interact with other medicines such as antibiotics and the oral

contraceptive pill, and it is best to inform the doctor and pharmacist about all of your medicines before starting new ones.
- She goes on to tell you that she is on the pill, but doesn't know which sort. Advise her to use an alternative form of contraceptive until she has had the opportunity to have a discussion with her GP.
- Moreover, tell her that if she does plan to have children it is worth telling the neurologist, who can ensure she is on the safest medication possible, as anticonvulsants can potentially affect the developing baby, leading to congenital defects.
- Briefly summarise the main discussion points from the consultation.
- Inform her that you will organise a further follow-up in the clinic in a few months' time.
- Ask if she has any other questions and close the interview.

Ethical issues

Confidentiality

See p. 7. Confidentiality is a cornerstone to the doctor–patient relationship. However, in certain situations (such as an epileptic who continues to drives vehicles despite medical advice to the contrary) confidentiality may be breached.

Driving

Refer to Appendix 1.

Epilepsy and pregnancy

Most anticonvulsants (particularly phenytoin, phenobarbital and carbamazepine) increase the risk of pregnancy in women on the oral contraceptive pill. In one study it was estimated that there was a 25-fold rise in the risk of pregnancy when an oral contraceptive was combined with phenytoin in comparison to those not taking phenytoin.

Generally speaking, it is recognised that women who suffer with epilepsy are more likely to have babies with birth defects in comparison to normal healthy controls. This is particularly true of women with poorly controlled epilepsy, resulting in frequent and severe fits during their pregnancy and also those in low socioeconomic groups. In addition to this, anticonvulsants may also cause congenital defects, which include developmental abnormalities of heart, face (e.g. cleft lip and palate), skull, limbs, abdominal organs and mental subnormality. It has been estimated that there is an approximately 1 per cent risk of birth defects with sodium valproate. Phenytoin and phenobarbitone can lead to vitamin K deficiency and bleeding diatheses in the newborn, who may require a vitamin K injection shortly after birth.

For these reasons, it is crucial that during pregnancy, women are given the smallest effective dose of anticonvulsants and are closely monitored.

Case 17: New diagnosis: ulcerative colitis

Candidate information

You are the SHO in a gastroenterology clinic.

Please read the scenario below. You may make notes on the paper provided. When the bell sounds enter the examination room to begin the consultation.

Patient: Mrs Elaine Winters

Age: 27 years

You review this geography teacher. She has previously been seen by your consultant, when she was referred with several months' history of bloody diarrhoea. A flexible sigmoido-scopy was arranged, which showed features of ulcerative colitis, and she was empirically commenced on a reducing course of prednisolone and mesalazine. The result from a biopsy taken at the time is now available and shows features strongly suggestive of moderately active ulcerative colitis. The diarrhoea is now settling on the medication. Your objective is to explain the diagnosis and the long-term management strategy.

You have 14 minutes to communicate with the patient followed by one minute for reflection before discussion with the examiners. You are not required to examine the patient.

Patient information

Mrs Elaine Winters

Aged 27 years

This 27-year-old geography teacher has suffered with bloody diarrhoea for several months and was seen in clinic a few weeks ago by a consultant. He had assessed her and had suggested that the problem may be an infection as the symptoms had started shortly after returning from a holiday in Sri Lanka. The other possibility was inflammatory bowel disease (IBD). Mrs Winters had not fully understood this term, but had not enquired further at the time. The doctor had arranged a 'camera test' as well as blood and stool tests, and a follow-up for today. Mrs Winters has never smoked and drinks alcohol infrequently. She lives with her husband. They have no children at present, but are trying for a baby. The only other medical problem she suffers with is an ongoing backache, for which she is taking an increasing amount of ibuprofen. She didn't mention this on the last occasion, but is keen to discuss it today. Her main concerns, however, relate to a recent discussion she had with her cousin, Mrs Tania Watts, who suffers with severe Crohn's disease and has had multiple operations including a colostomy. She had also suffered from severe side effects from steroid therapy, which included obesity, the development of osteoporosis and diabetes. Mrs Watts had told Mrs Winters that IBD was the same as Crohn's disease. Now she is extremely anxious that she will end up like her cousin. She is particularly worried about having a stoma bag and what impact the condition will have on her prospect for having children.

Possible prompts

- I don't understand what IBD means. Can you clarify this term please?
- My cousin has Crohn's disease. Is this the same condition?
- Can it be cured?
- Will I need to stay on the steroids for the rest of my life?
- Do I need an operation?
- Will changing my diet help at all?
- Is this an inherited condition?
- Will I be able to have children?

Possible interview plan

- Greet the lady and introduce yourself.
- Set the agenda. Confirm that she had previously seen your

consultant for bloody diarrhoea, and he had organised a series of investigations to find the cause for her problem.

- Enquire about her previous discussion in the clinic and what information had been given to her. She will probably say that she was told that she either had an infective illness or IBD.

- Ask her what this term means to her. She may volunteer that she has had a discussion with her cousin who suffers with Crohn's disease and that she is worried that she has the same problem.

- Explain to her that Crohn's disease is indeed one form of IBD or inflammatory bowel disease, but there are others. One of the other sorts is a condition called ulcerative colitis and say that the investigations are suggestive of ulcerative colitis as the cause for her illness. Elaborate by saying that colitis differs from Crohn's disease by affecting only the large bowel, whereas Crohn's can affect the whole length of the bowel. However, often it can be difficult to discriminate between the two conditions and the treatment for them is similar.

- She may raise concerns about her cousin and the operation she has had leading to a stoma and the possible side effects of steroid medication.

- Agree with her that these are potential complications of the illness, but reassure her that the vast majority of people with ulcerative colitis have a normal life without ever requiring an operation. Explain that steroid tablets (these are not to be confused with anabolic steroids that body builders use) are known to be the most effective therapy in the short term for difficult symptoms (which often include abdominal pain, bloody diarrhoea, fatigue and weight loss). Reassure her that even patients who are steroid-dependent (i.e. have flare-ups when they come off steroids) can be treated effectively with steroid-sparing drugs (such as azathioprine and methotrexate), which are less likely to have long-term side effects.

- Explain to her that some tablets such as ibuprofen and other non-steroidal anti-inflammatory drugs (NSAIDs) should be avoided in patients with colitis as it may cause an exacerbation of the condition and should be avoided.

- Reassure her that this disease is compatible with having children and is not inherited, although you are more likely to get the condition if you have a 'first-degree' relative who suffers with it.
- Tell her about the National Association for Crohn's and Colitis (NACC). This is a charitable organisation, which is a good source for information and self-help advice.
- Summarise the discussion and let her know that you will organise a follow-up in the clinic. Also give her contact details of your specialist IBD nurse and tell Mrs Winters to get in touch with her if her symptoms deteriorate.
- Thank her and close the interview.

Case 18: Obesity advice

Candidate information

You are the SHO in an endocrine clinic.

Please read the scenario below. You may make notes on the paper provided. When the bell sounds enter the examination room to begin the consultation.

Patient: Mrs Mary Sidebottom

Age: 44 years

This lady was referred to the clinic by her GP with a raised blood sugar, suspicious of diabetes. She normally runs a chip shop with her husband and generally leads a very sedentary lifestyle. She was reviewed by a consultant, who has diagnosed her with insulin resistance secondary to obesity. Endocrine causes for obesity have been excluded. The doctor had recommended weight loss by regular exercise and sticking to a calorie-controlled diet. Following her last clinic visit, an appointment was made for her to see a dietician. The dietician has reviewed her and given dietary advice, but did mention to the patient that there were drugs available that can help her to lose weight. Your objective is to discuss the patient's obesity and encourage her to lose weight. You must also answer any questions she has.

You have 14 minutes to communicate with the patient followed by one minute for reflection before discussion with the examiners. You are not required to examine the patient.

Patient information

Mrs Mary Sidebottom

Aged 44 years

This lady was found to have a raised blood sugar by her GP and was referred to a diabetologist for assessment. The consultant reviewed her and felt that it was related to her obesity. Mrs Sidebottom has always struggled with her weight, but it has escalated considerably over the last few years, particularly since opening a chip shop with her husband. In the past she tried various diets, but was unable to stick with them. She snacks throughout the day, which includes nibbling on the food in the chip shop, but because she doesn't have three regular meals, she feels that she hardly eats anything. Exercise has never been a part of Mrs Sidebottom's life and she rarely leaves her home. She has never cycled and doesn't know how to swim. The doctor who initially assessed her had referred her to a dietician. The dietician had given her information on calorie-controlled dieting, but also mentioned that there were tablets available to help people lose weight. Moreover, she also mentioned that operations could be done, which can lead to dramatic weight loss. With her lack of previous success with dieting the lady has not bothered to stick to the calorie-controlled diet prescribed for her. Instead, Mrs Sidebottom is very keen to explore the medical and surgical options. At the consultation today she intends to ask the doctor about the medicines available and the possible operations that can be performed.

Possible prompts

- Diets never seem to work for me.
- The dietician mentioned that there were tablets available to help people lose weight. Can I try these?
- What operations are available and would you be able to refer me for an operation?
- What's the Atkins diet? I hear that it is very effective.

Possible interview plan

- Greet the lady and introduce yourself.
- Set the agenda. Confirm that she was diagnosed with diabetes, which has been attributed to her weight and was advised to lose weight by exercise and diet. Ask how she is getting on and whether she has lost any weight.
- She will say that she has tried lots of diets and they have never worked and she is fed up of them. She may also add that she doesn't feel that she eats very much.
- Briefly take a dietary and exercise history. This is likely to confirm her sedentary lifestyle. She may be evasive about her intake so it is crucial that you ask about her exact intake and specifically ask about snack foods such as crisps, biscuits, fizzy drinks, chocolates and cakes. Ask about fresh fruit and vegetables.
- Reiterate that she must stick to a well-balanced, calorie-controlled diet and take regular exercise such as a brisk walk, which can be increased in intensity as her level of fitness increases. Emphasise the long-term benefits of losing weight, which will include reduced risk of heart disease, stroke and cancer. She must not assume that she is not eating very much, but instead keep a careful diary and attempt to adhere to her prescribed dietary regime.
- At this stage she is probably going to tell you about her conversation with the dietician who had told her about tablets that can help people lose weight.
- Agree with her that there are medications available that can potentially help people to lose weight, but they can only be used in people who are considered motivated and have exhausted other options. Moreover, the treatments are not without side effects and cannot be used indefinitely (see below).
- She may then ask about surgery as a means of treating obesity.
- Explain that surgical intervention is only carried out as a last resort if diet, exercise and medical management have been deemed to have failed. It can be very risky, with both anaesthetic and surgical risks.

- Summarise the discussion and explain to her that you will organise a follow-up appointment to ensure her progress is monitored.
- Ask if she has any other questions and close the interview.

NICE guidance

The National Institute of Clinical Excellence (NICE) has issued guidance on the use of surgery and drugs (sibutramine and orlistat) to help people lose weight. Full guidance is available on the NICE website. According to this guidance, these drugs can only be prescribed by hospital specialists, who should regularly review the patient. And then only if:

- diet and exercise have failed; or
- the patient's BMI is >27–28 with complications such as hypertension or diabetes; or
- the BMI >30.

Then they can only be continued beyond three months if there is documented weight loss.

Surgery may be considered when non-surgical strategies have failed. NICE recommends that surgery should only be offered:

- to patients who are >18 years
- where there are no contraindications to the surgery
- to patients who are fit for the surgery.

Case 19: The poorly compliant patient

Candidate information

You are an SHO in a chest clinic.

Please read the scenario below. You may make notes on the paper provided. When the bell sounds enter the examination room to begin the consultation.

Patient: Miss Rachel Robbins

Age: 24 years

This lady has had poorly controlled asthma for some years. She has been prescribed a beta agonist and a steroid inhaler. However, she has previously intimated that she does not like using the steroid inhaler and there is a suspicion that she doesn't use it at all. Your task is to discuss her compliance with her medication and advise her accordingly.

You have 14 minutes to communicate with the patient followed by one minute for reflection before discussion with the examiners. You are not required to examine the patient.

Patient information

Miss Rachel Robbins

Aged 24 years

This lady was diagnosed with mild asthma two years ago when she was started on a salbutamol inhaler. Her asthma was troublesome despite this and a year ago she had a steroid inhaler added to her prescription. However, about six months ago she read an article in a magazine highlighting the side effects of steroids, which had alarmed her, and now she rarely uses the steroid inhaler. She is particularly worried about weight gain, which was listed as a possible side effect. Miss Robbins is very conscious of her body image and frequently diets. She does not smoke. Her asthma is troublesome at present, particularly in the morning, but she attributes this to a change in the season and thinks that it will get better with time. She has now come to the clinic and is about to see one of the doctors.

Possible prompts

- My asthma is getting worse; I think it is because of the warm weather at the moment.
- I am worried about the steroids and their side effects and so don't like using my brown inhaler.

Possible interview plan

- Greet the lady and introduce yourself.
- Set the agenda. Confirm that she was diagnosed with asthma a few years ago and is being followed up in the clinic.
- Ask about her asthma symptoms and whether she feels they are deteriorating. She will reply in the affirmative and say that it is particularly bad in the morning. She will say that she suspects this is because of a change in the weather and it will probably get better with time.
- Ask her whether she uses the prescribed inhalers regularly and whether her technique has been reviewed.
- Her technique has been checked and she uses her blue inhaler regularly, but admits that she tends not to use the brown inhaler, as she is worried about side effects associated with steroid use, which she read about in a magazine. She is particularly worried about weight gain.
- Reassure her that only a tiny amount of steroid gets into her bloodstream from inhalation, and that this will have a negligible effect on her weight or cause any other systemic side effects. Conversely, it has a profound effect on reducing the inflammation within her lungs and would be a great help in helping with her asthma symptoms. Remind her that asthma can deteriorate and occasionally become life threatening and hence it is very important that we try and control it at an early stage. Also, it is worth emphasising

the point that when it does deteriorate, patients often have to start taking oral steroids and they can have the side effects she is concerned about.

- Ask her whether her views have changed at all and if she is likely to comply with her medication.
- If she agrees, then proceed; otherwise reiterate the above points before proceeding.
- Summarise the discussion. Explain that you will ask the asthma nurse to check on her in a few days' time and she should keep a record of her peak expiratory flow rates to ensure her asthma is improving.
- Ask if she has any other questions and close the interview.

Case 20: Counselling for an HIV test

Candidate information

You are an SHO on a medical ward.

Please read the scenario below. You may make notes on the paper provided. When the bell sounds enter the examination room to begin the consultation.

Patient: Mr Daniel Brown

Age: 27 years

This man was admitted with severe shortness of breath upon returning from a holiday in the Far East. Investigations show that he has Pneumocystis carinii *pneumonia, and is now making a good recovery with medication. You know from his history that he works as a bank clerk and lives with his mother. He drinks about 30 units of alcohol a week and smokes 10 cigarettes a day. He has confessed to 'experimenting' with drugs, although denies injecting them. He is a heterosexual male, but does not have a steady girlfriend. However, in the past he has had a number of casual and short-term relationships. Your task is to counsel him for an HIV test.*

You have 14 minutes to communicate with the patient followed by one minute for reflection before discussion with the examiners. You are not required to examine the patient.

Patient information

Mr Daniel Brown

Aged 27 years

This bank clerk was admitted to hospital with severe shortness of breath and he was subsequently diagnosed with *Pneumocystis carinii* pneumonia, which is being treated, and he is making a good recovery. The illness started shortly after return from holiday in Thailand. He smokes 10 cigarettes a day and drinks 30 units of alcohol per week. He lives with his mother and is not in a steady relationship. In the past he has experimented with drugs, but has never injected them. He is a heterosexual man and over the years he has had many short-term and casual relationships with unprotected sex. He has also on occasions used the services of prostitutes. He does not consider himself at high risk for developing HIV because he considers it a disease that affects homosexual men and those that abuse drugs with IV injections. He is about to see a doctor who will counsel him for an HIV test. Although initially Mr Brown will be reluctant, he will eventually come round to the idea of having the test.

Possible prompts

- What has my pneumonia got to do with HIV?
- Why should I undergo an HIV test? I'm not gay and have never injected myself with drugs.
- If I'm HIV positive, does that mean that I have AIDS?
- Will my mother be told of the result?
- Will my employers have to be informed?

Possible interview plan

- Greet the gentleman and introduce yourself.
- Set the agenda. Explain to him that you've come to speak to him regarding his recent diagnosis of a rare sort of pneumonia, which is often associated with an 'underactive' immune system. Ask him if he had any concerns regarding his immunity to infections and whether he was aware of any illnesses associated with poor immunity.
- If he says that he is aware of HIV or AIDS causing this problem, confirm his belief and proceed. Alternatively, explain that one cause of having a poor immune system and acquiring this rare respiratory tract infection was the human immunodeficiency virus (HIV).
- Wait for a response from him and briefly go into his perceived risk for acquiring HIV and his understanding of

this infection. He is likely to say that it is a condition that affects homosexual men and intravenous drug abusers.

- Explain to him that anybody can acquire this infection, which includes heterosexual men, particularly if they practise unprotected sex. And it is worth testing for as there is a very good therapy available and potentially it can prevent the infection passing on to others.
- Go on to explain that being HIV positive is not the same as having AIDS and briefly explain the difference. Tell him that the disease is less stigmatised these days, but being found positive may have implications for future employment and the prospect of obtaining health insurance.
- Explain that the test is carried out by obtaining a sample of blood from him and the result would be given to him in person. He must give his written consent before the test, and reassure him that the result will be treated with strict confidence.
- Ask him if he agrees to have the test or whether he would like more time to think it through and perhaps have another discussion.
- He is likely to agree to the test, in which case conclude by saying that you will obtain a consent form that he can sign before you proceed to the test.
- Thank him and conclude the interview.

Case 21: Man wanting to self-discharge

Candidate information

You are an SHO on call for the medical wards.

Please read the scenario below. You may make notes on the paper provided. When the bell sounds enter the examination room to begin the consultation.

Patient: Mr Nathan Charleston

Age: 41 years

This gentleman was admitted to hospital after an alcoholic binge and a benzodiazepine overdose. There had been no suicide note. At the time of admission, history taken from the patient's girlfriend suggests that the patient has been depressed for some time after the loss of his job and has frequently commented on taking his life and considered himself a failure. On the following day Mr Charleston has made a full medical recovery, but the team looking after him are very keen that he has a comprehensive psychiatric assessment. However, the gentleman, who is now alert and oriented, is adamant that he does not want to stay in hospital and will discharge himself. You have decided to speak with the gentleman to persuade him to stay in hospital until a psychiatrist has seen him.

You have 14 minutes to communicate with the patient followed by one minute for reflection before discussion with the examiners. You are not required to examine the patient.

Patient information

Mr Nathan Charleston

Aged 41 years

This gentleman was admitted to hospital the previous night after he had taken a large overdose of sleeping tablets (benzodiazepines) and a large amount of alcohol. The overdose had not been premeditated, but he had fantasised about taking his life for some months and had experienced problems with sleeping, occasionally finding it difficult to fall asleep and often waking up early in the morning. He had visited his GP, who was a little concerned about clinical depression, but had decided to initially try sleeping tablets and review him again to see how he was progressing. Mr Charleston's problems had started after he had lost his job as a highly paid marketing executive. He had been working in the same company for 22 years and considered himself extremely successful. Now his future looks bleak and he feels that he is a complete failure and has taken to drinking heavily. He was previously married and had one child, but the marriage broke down and ended up in divorce. He has been with his current girlfriend for nine months. Now, on the day after the overdose, he feels some remorse for his actions and generally fully recovered, and wants to leave the hospital. However, the medical team would like him to see a psychiatrist before he is discharged. Mr Charleston does not think that he is going mad and does not feel the need for a psychiatrist. One of the doctors looking after him will have a discussion and try to persuade him to stay. Although initially reluctant, Mr Charleston will finally agree to stay for psychiatric assessment.

Possible prompts

- No, I'm fine and I want to go home.
- Yes, I do regret my actions last night, but I don't I need to see a 'shrink'; I'm not mad.
- Yes, I have been feeling depressed of late – probably more so after losing my job.
- Well, I suppose it may be worth speaking with a psychiatrist.

Possible interview plan

- Greet the gentleman and introduce yourself.
- Set the agenda. Explain to him that you've decided to speak with him because you are worried about him discharging himself from the hospital before a psychiatrist has assessed him.
- Ask him why he wants to leave and not wait to be seen by a psychiatrist.
- He is likely to say that he regrets his actions and feels that he has made a full recovery and does not now want to stay in the hospital. Moreover, he does not think that he is mad and in need of a 'shrink'.
- Explain to him that the medical team do not think that he is mad, but are simply concerned that he has untreated depression and is likely to attempt suicide again. Go on to say that depression is considered a mental illness and there are very good therapies available.
- Ask him whether he feels that he is depressed and whether he has ever thought about ending his life, and could he see himself potentially benefiting from the help of a psychiatrist.
- He may go on to confirm that he is depressed and has had suicidal ideas and perhaps seeing the psychiatrist could benefit him. In this case congratulate him for staying and close the interview.

Alternatively:

- He may choose to ignore your advice and leave despite the consequences. You cannot keep him in hospital against his wishes and must allow him to leave, but ask him to sign a self-discharge note. You can come to a compromise by saying that you will refer him to the psychiatrist as an outpatient and asking whether he would be interested in attending. If he agrees, thank him and close the interview.

Suicide risk factors

- male sex
- older age, although there is a peak in adolescence

- psychiatric illness, e.g. depression, schizophrenia
- substance abuse
- diagnosis of serious and particularly chronic painful conditions
- life-altering events, e.g. loss of job
- bereavement
- past experiences, e.g. sexual abuse as child.

Case 22: Delay in review

Candidate information

You are an SHO in a cardiology clinic.

Please read the scenario below. You may make notes on the paper provided. When the bell sounds enter the examination room to begin the consultation.

Patient: Mr Ashok Shukla

Age: 57 years

This gentleman was admitted to hospital with severe chest pain and a subsequent coronary angiogram demonstrated triple-vessel disease, not appropriate for angioplasty. The cardiologist looking after him was concerned and explained that he could have a fatal heart attack if he didn't have prompt bypass surgery. Hence he would be referring him to one of the local cardiothoracic surgeons for an assessment soon as an outpatient. Today, three months later, Mr Shukla has arrived at the cardiology clinic and he is angry and upset that he still has not received an appointment to see one of the thoracic surgeons. Your task is to have a frank discussion with Mr Shukla regarding the delay in his treatment and how you intend to expedite his surgery.

You have 14 minutes to communicate with the patient followed by one minute for reflection before discussion with the examiners. You are not required to examine the patient.

Patient information

Mr Ashok Shukla

Aged 57 years

Mr Shukla was admitted to hospital three months previously with pains in his chest and a subsequent angiogram confirmed triple-vessel disease. At the time the cardiologist told him that he was at a significant risk of having a fatal heart attack and required prompt referral to a cardiothoracic surgeon (as an outpatient) for bypass surgery. However, three months later, Mr Shukla has still not received an appointment to see a surgeon. He is concerned that he will die before he has an operation and today at a follow-up cardiology clinic he fully intends to express his frustration and concerns to the doctor about to see him.

Possible prompts
- I am still getting chest pains and have not received an appointment to see a surgeon.
- It has been three months since my hospital admission and I am worried sick that I will drop dead before the appointment arrives.
- Will you be able to find out when they are likely to see me?

Possible interview plan
- Greet the patient and introduce yourself.
- Set the agenda. Confirm that this is a follow-up appointment and that he has previously been diagnosed with heart disease and is awaiting bypass surgery.
- Ask how the patent is getting on.
- Acknowledge the patient's disappointment with the delay in his treatment and allow him to vent his frustration. This could be a drawn-out process and the examiners will be keen to observe your skills that demonstrate empathy and rapport building as well as bargaining and negotiation.
- Explain that you too are disappointed with this delay and intend to rectify the situation by calling the surgical team and getting a date for the review before the man leaves today.
- Close the interview by asking the patient to wait outside while you get in contact with the surgical team and get a date for him. Alternatively, you can ask him to call you back and you will have a further management plan.

Government targets

The government set up *National Service Frameworks* (NSFs) in order to improve patient care and reduce inequalities in a series of identified priority areas, which includes the Coronary Heart Disease (CHD) NSF (published in 2000). This sets out a 10-year programme to transform the management of patients with heart disease and it has been estimated that as many as 20 000 lives a year should be saved.

As part of the modernisation of the NHS, the controversial *star ratings* were introduced to show how well an organisation is performing. For most trusts this is based on performance indicators, which are made up of four key targets:

- patient waiting times
- patient focus: patient's views on the trust
- clinical focus: outcomes after treatment such as surgery
- capacity and capability focus: trust resources, running and staff satisfaction.

Case 23: Obtaining consent for a specialist procedure

Candidate information

You are an SHO on call for medicine.

Please read the scenario below. You may make notes on the paper provided. When the bell sounds enter the examination room to begin the consultation.

Patient: Mrs Rahila Hussain

Age: 38 years

Mrs Hussain is a housewife with three small children. She is normally fit and well, but for the past few weeks she has suffered with a backache. She consulted her GP who prescribed ibuprofen tablets, which she has been taking with good result. However, earlier in the day she had an episode of frank haematemesis and passed some dark stools. Clinical examination has confirmed melaena and shows postural hypotension, but she is otherwise a well-looking woman. You are the RMO 'on call' overnight and she was 'handed over' to you by the admitting doctor. It is now 2am and you have just spoken with the endoscopist on call who feels that an urgent endoscopy is warranted, but to save time he would like you to consent her for the procedure. He explains that it is a very safe procedure with only a tiny risk of bleeding or perforation. Your task is to convey this information to the patient and, if you feel it is appropriate, obtain her consent.

You have 14 minutes to communicate with the patient followed by one minute for reflection before discussion with the examiners. You are not required to examine the patient.

Patient information

Mrs Rahila Hussain

Aged 38 years

Mrs Hussain is a housewife with three small children. She has suffered with a backache for some time now, which she attributes to lifting her children. A few weeks ago she asked her GP for advice and he prescribed her ibuprofen tablets, which she has been taking with good result. Earlier in the day she had passed some very dark stool, which looked like melaena, and later had vomited blood, which had prompted her to seek medical advice. The admitting doctor felt that she probably had an ulcer in her stomach and was going to organise an endoscopy and had put her nil by mouth. He has now gone off duty and one of his colleagues (the candidate) is going to speak with you about the procedure. Mrs Hussain is frustrated by her ordeal and the fact that it is the middle of the night and she has not had an endoscopy and not had any news as to when it is going to happen. She feels hungry and thirsty having been nil by mouth for so many hours. Above all she is worried about her three children.

Possible prompts

- How long will it be before I get my endoscopy?
- Will I be able to leave hospital tonight?
- Will I be able to eat and drink after the procedure?
- Do you think it was the ibuprofen tablets that caused the trouble?

Possible interview plan

- Greet the lady and introduce yourself.
- Set the agenda. Confirm that she was admitted to hospital within the last day with a suspected peptic ulcer bleed.
- Ask how she is feeling now.
- She is likely to be angry that she has not yet had her endoscopy test and is finding it very difficult being off food and water.

- Listen to her concerns empathetically and explain to her that often there is a delay in obtaining an endoscopic examination as it requires a specialist to perform the procedure and she should not worry about it being 2 o'clock in the morning as hospitals work round the clock. Further explain that although it is uncomfortable not to have any food for some hours, it is not likely to cause her any significant harm. It is, however, important that fluids are replaced and hence she is on a drip.
- Go on to say that you have spoken with the endoscopist on call and he will perform the endoscopy soon, but to save time has asked you to obtain consent from her. Explain that gastroscopy is a safe procedure, but there is a small risk of complication associated with perforation and bleeding. There are also complications associated with the sedation often used.
- She is likely to ask you about the degree of risk.
- Be very honest and say that you are not an expert in this area and couldn't comment on the details of the procedure, and perhaps she should have a chat with the endoscopist before going through the procedure.
- Say that you will document your discussion with her in the notes so that the endoscopist knows that he needs to obtain consent before proceeding to the gastroscopy.
- Summarise the discussion.
- Ask if she has any other questions and close the interview.

Case 24: Warfarin and the pregnant woman

Candidate information

You are an SHO in the haematology clinic.

Please read the scenario below. You may make notes on the paper provided. When the bell sounds enter the examination room to begin the consultation.

Patient: Mrs Patricia Murray

Age: 31 years

This lady was diagnosed with a large deep vein thrombosis (DVT) in her left leg three weeks previously and was commenced on warfarin. She has now presented to the anticoagulation clinic and has told the nurse that she has recently found out that she is pregnant. The nurse has asked you to speak with her to counsel her regarding the possible teratogenic effects of the drug and to come up with an alternative management strategy.

You have 14 minutes to communicate with the patient followed by one minute for reflection before discussion with the examiners. You are not required to examine the patient.

Patient information

Mrs Patricia Murray

Aged 31 years

Mrs Murray had presented to hospital three weeks previously with a swollen leg and had been diagnosed with a DVT. She had been commenced on warfarin and discharged from the hospital on the same day. One week ago she had found out that she was pregnant. She had previously had a period seven weeks ago. She has come to the anticoagulation clinic today and had told the nurse that she was pregnant. The nurse had looked alarmed, which concerned Mrs Murray, and had asked her to speak with one of the doctors in the clinic (the candidate). This pregnancy is very precious to Mrs Murray as she has been trying to have a baby with her partner for some years and they had even contemplated in vitro fertilisation (IVF). When the doctor explains the possible risks involved to both the baby and the pregnancy, Mrs Murray will become quite upset and somewhat angry. She will question why she had not been informed of the possible risks at the time she started the warfarin.

Possible prompts

- Is this serious?
- Is my baby going to be handicapped?
- Is this likely to increase my risk of miscarriage?
- Whose fault is this?
- Is there a chance that my pregnancy could still be normal?

Possible interview plan

- Greet the patient and introduce yourself.
- Confirm that a nurse has asked her to speak with you regarding her warfarin therapy, because she had found out that she was pregnant.
- Enquire what her understanding was regarding the use of warfarin in pregnancy and what additional information the nurse had given her.
- Listen attentively to her concerns and answer any immediate questions she may have.
- Apologise for her not being informed about the possible side effects of warfarin at the time of commencement. Confirm (if she is already aware) or explain that warfarin is a teratogenic drug, i.e. can cause birth defects and problems with pregnancy, such as bleeding and miscarriage. It is appropriate perhaps to only go into details of the sorts of defects that occur (see below) if she specifically asks about them.

- Give her a chance to respond and answer any queries. Listen carefully to her concerns and anxieties.
- Discuss future management plan, i.e. that you will be discussing the case with the consultant and can organise for Mrs Murray to speak with him also, if she has any further questions. Also explain that you will write to her obstetrician to ensure that she receives appropriate follow-up with them. Go on to tell her that she will probably need to go on to low molecular weight heparin injections until it is felt that her treatment is complete.
- Summarise the discussion and close.

Drug use in pregnancy

Drugs given during pregnancy can affect the developing foetus by producing a lethal, toxic, or teratogenic effect. Hence it is imperative that drugs are carefully reviewed before prescribing to pregnant women. Risks must also be assessed in any women of childbearing age and you must always assume that a woman is pregnant until there is evidence (or her word) to the contrary. The effect of any potential teratogenic agent is determined by the age of the foetus. The main period of organogenesis is between the 3rd and 8th weeks after conception, and teratogenesis is most likely at this stage. Commonly used drugs that may cause problems include various anticonvulsants, antibiotics and anti-coagulants. Warfarin (coumarin) is known to be teratogenic. Effects on the foetus include saddle nose, frontal bossing, short stature, midface hypoplasia, cardiac defects, blindness and mental retardation. Warfarin should be avoided during the first trimester. It should also be avoided around the time of delivery and unfractionated or more conveniently low molecular weight heparin provide a safer alternative where anticoagulation is needed.

Case 25: Withdrawal of consent

Candidate information

You are an SHO working on a liver unit in a large teaching hospital.

Please read the scenario below. You may make notes on the paper provided. When the bell sounds enter the examination room to begin the consultation.

Patient: Mr Tom Waters

Age: 53 years

This gentleman has been followed up as an outpatient for one year with abnormal liver biochemistry. He is obese and known to drink alcohol excessively, and has arrived today to undergo a liver biopsy to investigate this further. Consent for the procedure had previously been obtained at the outpatient clinic. Potential risks such as bleeding, pneumothorax, pain and failure to obtain liver tissue had been discussed and documented in the notes. He was also given a leaflet to take away with him giving full details of the procedure. Although he has arrived at the department, he is concerned about the safety of the procedure and not proceeding with it. To discuss things further he has asked to speak to a doctor. The registrar, who normally performs the procedure, is busy on the liver ITU and has asked you to talk with the patient. Your objective is to discuss the patient's concerns and to ascertain whether or not he wishes to proceed with the procedure.

You have 14 minutes to communicate with the patient followed by one minute for reflection before discussion with the examiners. You are not required to examine the patient.

Patient information

Mr Tom Waters

Aged 53 years

This gentleman is overweight and has been drinking 60 units of alcohol per week for many years. He was admitted to hospital with abdominal pain, which was thought to be gastritis. But blood tests showed deranged liver biochemistry and hence he was referred to a hepatologist for an opinion. The initial liver screen proved normal and hence it was decided to proceed to a liver biopsy, which was discussed with Mr Waters at the previous clinic visit by a consultant. He mentioned potential risks associated with the procedure such as: bleeding, perforation of bowel, pain, pneumothorax and failure to obtain liver tissue. Then he had arranged a date for the procedure and sent the gentleman away with a leaflet to read at his leisure. During the previous evening, Mr Waters had got round to reading the leaflet and was horrified to find out that there was a significant risk of death associated with the procedure. He had difficulty going to sleep overnight and now, after arriving at the department, would like to discuss the procedure again before making his mind up. He will directly question the interviewing doctor and ask him about his experience of liver biopsies. During the course of the discussion, Mr Waters makes his mind up and is adamant that he does not want to undergo the liver biopsy procedure.

Possible prompts

- I read that you can die after having this procedure?
- How bad is the pain after the procedure?
- How many liver biopsies have you carried out?
- I refuse to have the procedure. What will happen now?

Possible interview plan

- Greet the patient and introduce yourself.
- Set the agenda. Confirm that he has asked to speak with a doctor because he is concerned about the liver biopsy procedure.

- Ask him what specific concerns he has. He will say that he is worried about all the side effects, but reading the leaflet that was given to him shows that there is a significant risk of death. Also, he is not keen on a procedure that can be very painful.
- Agree with him that there is a small risk of death, but the procedure is necessary to investigate the cause of his liver disease. The pain, which is often referred to the shoulder, can be troublesome in a small minority of patients. Most patients suffer very little pain and have analgesics prescribed.
- At this stage Mr Waters will ask you if you have ever carried out any liver biopsies and what experience you have of them.
- Explain to him honestly that you have had very little experience of them (unless of course you have had lots of experience!), but you can organise for him to speak with a doctor who routinely performs the procedure.
- Mr Waters will have made his mind up and decide that he does not want to have the procedure and wants to leave the hospital soon.
- Say that you will inform your seniors of his decision.
- Thank him and close the interview.

The liver biopsy

The liver biopsy needs to be carried out for a wide variety of conditions affecting the liver. This is particularly true when there are diagnostic uncertainties and further management strategies need to be based on the results of the liver biopsy. However, there is a significant mortality associated with the technique (at around 0.1 per cent, usually secondary to haemorrhage) and hence it should not be undertaken lightly. Moreover, there is morbidity associated with the procedure, the most common of which is pain (at around 30 per cent). The safety of the procedure can be optimised by performing the procedure either during an ultrasound scan or having had one recently. Also, most authorities agree that prior to the procedure the platelet count should be greater than $60\,000/mm^3$ and prothrombin time less than 4 seconds prolonged.

Consent

Refer to p. 2. But essentially, a procedure cannot be carried out on a competent adult without their consent.

Case 26: Worried about infection after blood transfusion

Candidate information

You are the medical SHO 'on call'.

Please read the scenario below. You may make notes on the paper provided. When the bell sounds enter the examination room to begin the consultation.

Patient: Miss Emma Rutledge

Age: 19 years

This lady presented to hospital with abdominal pain and was diagnosed with a ruptured ovarian cyst that had bled profusely and caused a drop in her haemoglobin. She was adequately resuscitated (which included a blood transfusion with three units of blood) and taken to theatre where emergency surgery was performed. Now she is five days post procedure and has made a good recovery and is nearly ready to be discharged from the obstetrics and gynaecology ward. However, she told the discharging doctor that she is concerned about the blood transfusion she received. She is particularly worried about the long-term prospect of having acquired an infection. The SHO looking after her has asked you to speak with her. Your objective is to listen to her concerns and if possible to reassure her.

You have 14 minutes to communicate with the patient followed by one minute for reflection before discussion with the examiners. You are not required to examine the patient.

Patient information

Miss Emma Rutledge

Aged 19 years

This English literature student presented to hospital with abdominal pain and was found to have a ruptured ovarian cyst, which had required surgical intervention. Prior to the operation she had received three units of blood. Previously she had been fit and well and not on any regular medication. Now, five days postoperatively, she had made a good recovery and is ready to be discharged from hospital. However, she is concerned about infection risk associated with the blood transfusion. In particular she is concerned about hepatitis, as her sister had developed jaundice after returning from a holiday in India. At that time the doctors had enquired about blood transfusions and had explained that there was a risk of developing hepatitis after receiving a blood transfusion. She is also aware that HIV can be transmitted through blood. Miss Rutledge had raised her concerns to the doctor looking after her. But he felt unable to answer her questions and has instead referred her to the medical SHO, who is about to see her.

Possible prompts
- I'm worried about a risk of developing an infection from contaminated blood.
- My sister developed hepatitis after a holiday and the doctor said that people could get hepatitis infections through a blood transfusion.
- Is there a chance that I could contract HIV from this transfusion?
- How can I be sure I haven't got these diseases?

Possible interview plan
- Greet the lady and introduce yourself.
- Set the agenda. Confirm that she has asked to speak with a doctor because she is worried about the blood transfusion.
- Ask about specific concerns that she may have. She is likely

to go into details about her concerns regarding HIV and hepatitis infections.

- Reassure her that blood and blood products are tested for hepatitis and HIV infections and it is highly unlikely that these viruses would contaminate the blood she received.
- She may say that she remains concerned and ask if there is a way to be certain.
- Explain to her that she could have HIV and hepatitis tests. But there needs to be a three-month gap between the potential exposure and testing, as it takes that long for the antibodies to become positive in the blood. However, she would have to see a counsellor before a test could be carried out, as particularly being HIV positive has serious long-term implications for a patient. Of course, in the unlikely event of her being found to be positive for one of these viruses, it would be a moot point as to whether she acquired the infection before or after the blood transfusion.
- Summarise the discussion and ask if she has any more questions.
- Close the interview.

Case 27: Patient requesting cannabis

Candidate information

You are a medical SHO in a clinic.

Please read the scenario below. You may make notes on the paper provided. When the bell sounds enter the examination room to begin the consultation.

Patient: Ms Helen Cummings

Age: 49 years

This lady has suffered with long-standing severe back pain for a number of years and has tried numerous medications and aids (such as a 'TENS' machine) with only limited benefit. She has been extensively investigated and reviewed by both a pain specialist and an orthopaedic surgeon, who could not find an obvious cause to explain the pain. At present, she is taking codeine and paracetamol and is complaining of severe constipation. She has come to the follow-up clinic today to discuss further options to relieve her pain. In particular, she wants to discuss the possibility of cannabis being prescribed for her pain. Your task is to discuss this and other treatment options with her.

You have 14 minutes to communicate with the patient followed by one minute for reflection before discussion with the examiners. You are not required to examine the patient.

Patient information

Ms Helen Cummings

Aged 49 years

This lady has suffered with back pain for many years. She has previously been investigated – including an appointment with the orthopaedic surgeons – and no obvious cause was ever found. Over the years she has tried numerous medications and alternative therapies such as acupuncture and a 'TENS' machine with only limited benefit. She is currently on paracetamol and a high dose of codeine phosphate, which does give her pain relief, but she tends to get very constipated and has to take laxatives regularly. A few weeks ago she saw a television programme that followed a group of patients with intractable pain and it had demonstrated the benefits of cannabis (and drugs derived from the plant) in the management of pain symptoms. Ms Cummings had got very excited by this programme and is very keen to explore this option at the clinic visit today.

Possible prompts

- My pain is reasonably controlled but I suffer with awful constipation.
- I saw a television programme about the use of cannabis in patients with pain symptoms like mine. Is that something you can prescribe for me?

Possible interview plan

- Greet the patient and introduce yourself.
- Set the agenda. Confirm that she is being followed up in the clinic as she has ongoing back pain.
- Ask her how she is getting on. She will tell you that she still suffers with the back pain, but the medication affords her some relief. But she is very troubled with constipation when she takes the codeine. However, she is able to open her bowels with the aid of laxatives.
- Explain that the constipation is a well-recognised side effect of opiate drugs like codeine. And you can do one of two things:
  - either persist with the current regime and use laxatives as required, or
  - you will discuss the case with your consultant and decide whether there needs to be a change in medication. But you note that she has used numerous medications without benefit.

- At this point she may tell you about a television programme she has seen where people with intractable pain were using cannabis with good result. And she asks you whether this is something that she would be able to try.
- Explain to her that while there is some anecdotal evidence for cannabis as a treatment in various medical conditions, including pain, there is no clinical proof for its use. Moreover, the drug is not licensed for clinical use (indeed remains an illegal substance) and is only used in clinical trials.
- She agrees to stay on her current treatment, but would like to be followed up in the clinic.
- Ask her if she has any other concerns or questions.
- If she does not, thank her and close the interview.

Cannabis

The legal position

Cannabis was first declared illegal in the UK in 1928 following the Dangerous Drugs Act. It primarily outlawed private use, but allowed medical use. The United Nations Single Convention on Narcotic Drugs 1961 failed to recognise any medical indications for the drug and in 1971, the Misuse of Drugs Act made possession and supply unlawful. At the time of writing cannabis and its derivatives are not licensed for use for any medical condition in the UK.

In January 2004, cannabis was reclassified from a Class B to a Class C drug. Put simply this means that the drug remains illegal, but you are less likely to go to prison for possession and, more importantly, supply of the drug. At the present time, there are a number of cases working their way through the courts to establish the legal position of the defence of 'medical necessity' used by people who supply cannabis only for symptom relief to people with chronic medical conditions such as multiple sclerosis.

Medicinal use

The drug is obtained from the plant *Cannabis sativa*, which has been used for medicinal purposes for many centuries. Its uses have included the treatment of asthma, nausea, pain, muscular spasms and as a sleep aid. Although there is considerable interest, at present there is no absolute clinical evidence, which proves that cannabis is beneficial in any of these conditions except perhaps nausea and vomiting.

Perhaps the greatest interest is in cannabis and its active derivatives (particularly delta-9 tetrahydrocannabinol – THC) in the treatment of multiple sclerosis. The largest study to date was the CAMS (Cannabis in MS) trial, which was coordinated from Plymouth and funded by the Medical Research Council, and published in November 2003. It was a randomised, controlled, double-blind trial involving 660 patients. Patients were randomly allocated to one of the following groups:

- cannabis extract (Cannador) – standardised to contain 2.5 mg THC
- dronabinol (Marinol) – synthetic THC
- placebo.

Then they were followed up for a total of 15 weeks initially and enrolled into the extension trial. Although patients subjectively noted an improvement in their spasticity and mobility, objective measures (such as the Ashworth scale) failed to show significant improvement.

Case 28: Recruiting a patient into a clinical trial

Candidate information

You are the medical SHO in a gastroenterology clinic.

Please read the scenario below. You may make notes on the paper provided. When the bell sounds enter the examination room to begin the consultation.

Patient: Mr Hugh Trotter

Age: 36 years

This gentleman has been referred by his GP with persistent symptoms of gastro-oesophageal reflux, despite treatment with antacids and H2 antagonists. A gastroscopy was carried out, which shows moderate oesophagitis. Your consultant has reviewed his notes and has asked you to start him on a proton pump inhibitor (PPI). However, he is conducting a clinical trial at present comparing the efficacy of PPI A versus PPI B for symptomatic relief of reflux symptoms and is keen for you to recruit this patient into the study. The study protocol simply involves randomly starting either PPI A or B and then for the patient to complete a postal questionnaire in two months time. Your objective is to have a discussion with this gentleman and if possible recruit him into the study.

You have 14 minutes to communicate with the patient followed by one minute for reflection before discussion with the examiners. You are not required to examine the patient.

Patient information

Mr Hugh Trotter

Aged 36 years

This gentleman has suffered with heartburn and dyspepsia for about 12 months. He initially saw his GP, who prescribed him an antacid, which proved useless. The GP then prescribed an H2 antagonist and despite this and lifestyle advice (lose weight, not to eat late at night, raise the head of the bed) his symptoms persisted and he was finally referred to the hospital and has subsequently had a gastroscopy performed. He wasn't told the result of this, but instead had a follow-up appointment to which he has come to today. The doctor he is about to see will suggest that he goes on a PPI. However, the doctor will attempt to recruit Mr Trotter into a clinical trial comparing the efficacy of two PPIs (A and B) in the management of gastro-oesophageal reflux disease. Although, the gentleman will carefully consider taking part in the clinical trial, in the end he will decline.

Possible prompts
- Did they find the cause of my symptoms?
- What does the term oesophagitis mean?
- Is there treatment available for reflux disease?
- Do I have to take part in the clinical trial?
- What advantage is there for me?
- If I decline to take part, will that count against me in the future?

Possible interview plan
- Greet the patient and introduce yourself.
- Set the agenda. Confirm that he was referred by his GP because of his symptoms of heartburn and subsequently had a gastroscopy performed.
- Explain that the gastroscopy and the symptoms are strongly suggestive of acid reflux disease, which has caused inflammation of the gullet. Explain this in simple, lay terms

without using any complex medical jargon and check with him that he understands.

- Go on to explain that an effective treatment for this condition is use of drugs that reduce the amount of acid in the stomach known as proton pump inhibitors and that we need to start one of these drugs. Confirm that he understands this.
- Now, further explain that the department is currently conducting an experiment where the strength of one acid-reducing drug is being compared with another. And that you would like to enrol him into a trial, which is being supervised by your consultant, comparing one drug with another. Say to him that you would like to enrol him into this trial, but his consent is required.
- At this point he may enquire whether he is obliged to enrol into this study and whether he is likely to be discriminated against if he does not, i.e. would he still get optimum treatment.
- Reassure him that his treatment would not be affected by whether he decides to enrol into the study.
- He will say to you that he does not wish to take part in the study and would simply like to be treated for his condition.
- Reassure him that you will start him on a proton pump inhibitor and arrange a follow-up appointment to ensure that his symptoms are improving.
- Ask him if he has any further questions.
- If he does not, thank him and close the interview.

Research and ethics

See p. 16.

Case 29: The aggressive patient

Candidate information

You are the SHO on a diabetes ward.

Please read the scenario below. You may make notes on the paper provided. When the bell sounds enter the examination room to begin the consultation.

Patient: Mr Lance Riddell

Age: 49 years

The nurse looking after Mr Riddell has asked you to speak with him because of his behaviour earlier in the day. At lunchtime, he had become very aggressive towards the auxiliary nurse serving food. He had been verbally abusive and had threatened to hit her. The young nurse involved had been very upset. Mr Riddell had finally calmed down after security had been called to the ward. Prior to this episode the gentleman had been well behaved. He is a known insulin-dependent diabetic, who is being treated for an ulcer on his foot. Your task is to have a discussion with Mr Riddell and explain to him that abusive behaviour will not be tolerated.

You have 14 minutes to communicate with the patient followed by one minute for reflection before discussion with the examiners. You are not required to examine the patient.

Patient information

Mr Lance Riddell

Aged 49 years

This gentleman is known to suffer with insulin-dependent diabetes mellitus and is in hospital receiving treatment for a nasty foot ulcer. One of the doctors looking after him is about to speak with him regarding an incident that took place earlier in the day. At lunchtime he was feeling very hungry and the nurse serving food had walked past him twice without serving his dinner. This had caused him to become agitated and eventually he had lost his temper and shouted at her and had threatened to hit her. Security officers were called to the ward (which Mr Riddell had thought unnecessary) and the gentleman had calmed down. This behaviour is out of character for him and he regrets his action. He thinks that he may have been hypoglycaemic, which tends to make him temperamental. When he speaks with the doctors he will express his remorse.

Possible prompts

- I'm sorry I was aggressive at lunchtime.
- I would like to apologise to the nurse.
- I suspect it was low blood sugar that caused me to behave in this manner.

Possible interview plan

- Greet the patient and introduce yourself.
- Set the agenda. Tell him that you have been asked to speak with him regarding his behaviour at lunchtime.
- Ask him to tell you his side of the story. He will explain to you that he felt agitated at lunchtime, which escalated when the food trolley had gone past him twice, without him being served. He attributes his actions to a possible episode of hypoglycaemia.
- Ask him if he has any animosity towards the nurse in question and whether this behaviour was out of character for him. Also enquire if he feels that the nurse had purposefully failed to serve him food. If there is no intentional animosity on either side, proceed.
- Ask him if he regrets his actions and whether he would like to apologise to the nurse he was aggressive towards.
- If he does regret his actions then reassure him that the matter does not need to be taken any further and he will be

given the opportunity to apologise to the nurse in question, provided this is acceptable to her.
- Ask him if there are other concerns.
- If not, thank him and close the interview.

Managing aggressive patients

Unfortunately, verbal and occasionally physical aggression against NHS staff is not uncommon. To combat this, the government and the profession have agreed on zero tolerance towards aggression. The NHS Zero Tolerance Zone is a nation-wide campaign initiative to reinforce this policy. As part of this policy all trusts must develop a policy to tackle aggression against staff, which should include a policy on withholding or withdrawing treatment from repetitively violent and aggressive patients. This should only be carried out when warnings have failed. If the situation is serious, the police may have to be involved.

Case 30: The near miss: discussion with the patient

(Review this case with case 49: The near miss: discussion with nurse)

Candidate information

You are a medical SHO working on a chest ward.

Please read the scenario below. You may make notes on the paper provided. When the bell sounds enter the examination room to begin the consultation.

Patient: Mr John Powell

Age: 39 years

This gentleman has asked to speak with you to complain about a near miss, which could have been potentially fatal. He is known to suffer with asthma and is currently on the ward recovering from an attack. He has been commenced on oral prednisolone. He is known to have a severe allergy to aspirin, which has previously resulted in an ITU admission because of laryngeal oedema. This morning the nurse administering the drugs had got her prescription sheets mixed up and given him aspirin, which was intended for the patient in the next bed. He had spotted the mistake and scolded the nurse and demanded to speak with a doctor. Your objective is to have a discussion with Mr Powell regarding this error and how you plan to proceed.

You have 14 minutes to communicate with the patient followed by one minute for reflection before discussion with the examiners. You are not required to examine the patient.

Patient information

Mr John Powell

Aged 39 years

This gentleman is in hospital recovering from a severe attack of asthma. He is on oral prednisolone and is making a good recovery. Mr Powell is known to have a severe allergy to aspirin, which has previous required admission to the ITU with laryngeal oedema. This morning the nurse on the drug round had inadvertently given him aspirin (intended for another patient) instead of his prednisolone tablets. Luckily he had spotted the mistake in time and had avoided a potential disaster. He had scolded the nurse and demanded to speak with a doctor, who is about to see him now. Mr Powell will relay his concerns to the doctor and demand that some sort of action is taken against the nurse who he holds responsible.

Possible prompts

- I'm very upset by this mistake.
- I could have died because of this.
- How can I be sure it will not happen again?

Possible interview plan

- Greet the patient and introduce yourself.
- Set the agenda. Confirm that he has asked to speak with a doctor regarding an incident with his medication.
- Briefly ask him to relay the incident and his specific concerns. He will tell you about the mix-up with the tablets, which could have resulted in a life-threatening emergency.
- Ask him whether the nurse had verified his identification (either verbally or by checking his wristband) prior to administering the drug.
- Reassure him that you will speak with both the nurse involved and the sister on the ward to investigate the matter further, and tell the consultant looking after him about the mistake. Moreover, you will ensure that a clinical incident form is completed and further action taken as necessary.

- Ask him if he has any further questions or concerns.
- If he does not, thank him and close the interview.

Clinical governance in a 'nutshell'

The concept was first introduced by the Department of Health (DoH) in 1997 in response to public concerns about access to, and quality of, healthcare in different parts of the country. The chief executive takes ultimate responsibility for clinical governance and the Healthcare Commission (CHAI, formerly known as the Commission for Health Improvements, CHI) will assess every trust and primary care trust (PCT) to review clinical governance arrangements. Clinical governance is about having mechanisms in place to deliver the best-quality care within the NHS. This is done through the following key aspects.

Quality standards

Professional bodies and the National Service Frameworks (NSFs) can develop standards and milestones for service improvements both locally and nationally, while the merits of individual drugs and treatments are being assessed by The National Institute for Clinical Excellence (NICE). Through clinical audit, healthcare professionals can compare their practice with these agreed standards. It is important for doctors and other health professionals to continually develop their practices by using an evidence-based approach and by continued professional development.

Risk management

Many adverse incidents are potentially preventable. Risk management is a proactive approach, which identifies the risks that exist, and attempts to eliminate them. A crucial element is to learn from experience of adverse events. Lessons can be learned from:

- clinical incident reporting
- near misses
- complaints from patients, families and caregivers.

Patient satisfaction

An important aspect to this is the Patient Advice and Liaison Services (PALS), which should be available in all trusts and provide confidential advice and support to patients, families and their carers.

Case 31: Herbal therapy for angina

Candidate information

You are an SHO in a cardiology clinic.

Please read the scenario below. You may make notes on the paper provided. When the bell sounds enter the examination room to begin the consultation.

Patient: Mrs Jasmine McBride

Age: 52 years

This 52-year-old librarian has been referred by her GP with intermittent chest pains. An exercise tolerance test previously carried out had demonstrated ECG changes consistent with a diagnosis of angina. The GP had commenced her on aspirin, a beta-blocker and a sublingual nitrate. The lady had refused to take the prescribed medication because she is a firm believer in holistic medicine. Your task today is to have a discussion with her and persuade her to take her conventional medicines.

You have 14 minutes to communicate with the patient followed by one minute for reflection before discussion with the examiners. You are not required to examine the patient.

Patient information

Mrs Jasmine McBride

Aged 52 years

This lady presented to her GP with chest pains. She was very reluctant to see him, but had been persuaded to go by her husband and teenage sons. He had organised an exercise tolerance test, and on the basis of this had confidently diagnosed angina secondary to ischemic heart disease (IHD), which can deteriorate and result in a heart attack. Mrs McBride understands that angina is caused by reduced blood flow to the heart muscle.

A prescription for various medicines (aspirin, a beta-blocker and a sublingual nitrate) had been issued, but Mrs McBride had refused to take them because she is a firm believer in holistic, and particularly, herbal medicine. Her interest in 'alternative medicine' had started some years previously when her sister had developed breast cancer and the doctors were unable to save her. She had died a horrible agonising death and after that time Mrs McBride's faith in conventional medicine had ceased. Most of her knowledge of alternative therapies comes from her research into the subject on the Internet. Today she has come to the hospital, again at her husband's request, and is rather reluctant to be here. The doctor in the clinic will try to persuade her, but despite his best efforts, Mrs McBride will refuse to start taking the prescribed medicines, instead preferring to take her herbal remedies. She will, however, agree to come back to the clinic in due course.

Possible prompts

- Yes, I understand that I have angina and I know this is caused by reduced blood flow to the heart.
- I believe that holistic and herbal remedies are much more effective than what you can offer me at the hospital.
- Your medicines didn't do my sister any good; she died in agony of breast cancer.
- I've seen lots of evidence for the effectiveness of herbal remedies in books and on the Internet.
- Yes I do know that angina can lead to a heart attack, but I think my medicines will prevent this happening.
- I am happy to come back to the clinic again.

Possible interview plan

- Greet the patient and introduce yourself.
- Set the agenda. Confirm that she has been referred by her GP because of diagnosis of angina.
- Ask her what she understands about her diagnosis. She will

tell you that it is pain secondary to a reduced blood flow to the heart.

- Tell her that you understand that the GP had started her on some medicines in an attempt to treat the angina, but she had refused to take them.
- Ask her to tell you the reason for this (perhaps it is better not to put this in terms of non-compliance). She will tell you that she prefers holistic/complementary medicine. She may choose to tell you the reason for this, inasmuch as the failure of conventional therapy to treat her sister, who died in agony through breast cancer.
- Say that while there is good evidence that complementary therapy can be effective in a wide variety of conditions, you are not aware of any evidence that advocates its sole use in ischemic heart disease. On the other hand there is much evidence and experience in the use of conventional drug therapies in the treatment of this condition and therefore it is important that she takes the prescribed medications.
- She will choose to disagree and say that she has seen lots of evidence on the Internet, which validates the use of herbal treatments in angina therapy.
- Ask her if she realises that angina can deteriorate and can lead to a heart attack. She will tell you that she does, but does not expect her condition to deteriorate as she is treating it appropriately.
- Say that you respect her wishes and will not press the point, but will arrange for her to be followed up in clinic. She will say that she does not mind this and agree to come back to the clinic.
- Thank her for coming to the clinic today and close the interview.

Alternative/complementary therapy

Although most of these treatments have been around for a very long time, they have only become popular in the West over the last 30–40 years. They consist of a heterogeneous group of therapies that are often viewed with scepticism and suspicion by doctors. Also included are a wide variety of disparate disciplines that exist largely outside conventional, hospital-based medical practice. Many alternative therapies (such as acupuncture, chiropractic therapy, hypnotherapy and nutritional therapy) are becoming an accepted part of healthcare practice. But others (such as reflexology, reiki, yoga, etc.) remain very much on the fringe of our practice. One of the reasons why doctors do not readily use complementary therapy is because of the lack of scientific evidence. Research tends not to be carried out on these treatments for a number of reasons, which include the following.

Funding and facilities

First, there is little or no funding, particularly as there is no commercial interest for pharmaceutical companies to invest in complementary medicine. Moreover, generally speaking, complementary practitioners have no training in critical evaluation of existing research or practical research skills and have a lack of an academic infrastructure, which means limited access to, for instance, computer and library facilities.

Difficulty in data interpretation

Because of the nature of these treatments, it is very difficult to isolate the individual component, which may be responsible for the favourable end result. Take for example herbal remedies – these tend to be concoctions made up of many individual drugs and it is often impossible to know what the effective component is.

Regulation

Another problem faced by complementary practitioners is the lack of regulation. Apart from osteopaths and chiropractors, practitioners are not obliged to join any official register before setting up in practice. For this reason they are often perceived as 'quacks', who are not qualified to give a professional opinion. However, the climate is changing and many practitioners are now members of appropriate registering or accrediting bodies.

Internet therapy

The Internet is often used as a powerful source of medical information. There are many very useful sites out there and it's not unusual for medical practioner's to direct patients to specific sites for more information on their particular conditions and ideas for self-help. However, for patients, the sheer size of the 'World Wide Web' makes it a difficult task to isolate the helpful information and they run the risk of being misguided. The problem is that most of the *medical* information on the Internet is not put there by medical practitioners, but instead by well-meaning individuals or *self-help* groups and, unfortunately, often by charlatans, whose sole objective is to make money from people seeking a medical solution.

Discussions with relatives

Case 32: Stroke and resuscitation decision

Candidate information

You are the RMO on-call at a busy district general hospital.

Please read the scenario below. You may make notes on the paper provided. When the bell sounds enter the examination room to begin the consultation.

Subject: Mrs Una Watkins

Age: 46 years

Re: father, Mr Arthur Whiteman, aged 78 years

You have just finished reviewing Mr Arthur Whiteman, who is a 78-year-old man brought to hospital unconscious. Subsequent clinical examination and CT scan of the head have confirmed a massive stroke. You have discussed the case with the consultant on call and his feeling is that this man is not likely to survive the night and should be for 'TLC', and not for resuscitation. The man's daughter (Mrs Una Watkins) is very keen to speak with you about her father's illness. Your objective is to convey the poor prognosis and to discuss the resuscitation status.

You have 14 minutes to communicate with the subject followed by one minute for reflection before discussion with the examiners.

Subject information

Mrs Una Watkins

Aged 46 years

Re: father, Mr Arthur Whiteman, aged 78 years

This lady's father, Mr Arthur Whiteman (aged 78 years), was admitted to hospital after he collapsed at home and became unconscious. He has not regained consciousness since. Normally he is a fit and well man who occasionally smokes a pipe and drinks a few pints of mild each week. He is a widower, lives alone and is self-caring. Mrs Watkins has always been close to her father and checks on him on a daily basis and this sudden collapse has come as a great surprise for her. She is about to speak with a doctor who has admitted her father and will be horrified to hear that he has had a massive stroke and is not likely to recover from this. Prior to this interview, she will have no idea as to why he suddenly collapsed. She will find it hard to accept the medical decision that her father should not be resuscitated if his heart stops beating. Her father had never made a living will/ advanced directive, but she recalls that when her mother was dying with terminal cancer he had said that if his time ever came he would not want any 'messing around'. Upon reflection, she feels that he would prefer to die with dignity if there was no real chance of reasonable recovery.

Possible prompts

- Will Dad get better?
- Is he going to die?
- He's always been very active and in good health. Why has this happened so suddenly?
- Is he in pain?
- Is there nothing you can do for him?
- Will you stop all the treatment?

Possible interview plan

- Greet the subject and introduce yourself to her.

- Set the agenda. Confirm with her that she has asked to speak with you regarding her father's condition.
- Ask her what she knows about the cause of her father's illness and how he is getting on.
- She will not know the cause of her father's collapse or have any idea of his prognosis. However, it is important that you listen to her both carefully and empathetically, and without too much interruption.
- Explain to her in plain English that the clinical examination and the CT scan show that her father has suffered a massive stroke. Pause and let her absorb this information.
- Go on to explain that it is unlikely that he will regain consciousness and in all probability he is likely to deteriorate and die. It is especially important that you pause and let her comprehend this information.
- She may ask you how much time he has before he dies. Be honest and say that it is difficult to predict, but given the severity of the stroke it will probably be in the next 24 hours (there must be absolutely no mention of crystal balls or pieces of string!).
- Carefully breach the subject of resuscitation. Explain to her that you have discussed her father's case with a consultant physician and he feels that it would be futile to attempt cardiopulmonary resuscitation and that it is best that he is declared not-for-resuscitation.
- Ask her if the patient had ever expressed an opinion on this subject or whether she was aware of a living will that he had left. She may tell you that when her mother was terminally ill he had said that if he were ever in a similar position then he would not like to be 'messed about'. So, in her opinion, he probably would not want to be resuscitated and instead die with some dignity.
- Reassure her that in the unlikely event of her father making any sort of recovery, the resuscitation decision would be reviewed. And even though he is not for resuscitation his basic medical and nursing care will not be affected.
- Ask her if she has any other concerns or questions.
- If not, thank her and close the interview.

Ethical issues

For a discussion on CPR and other 'end-of-life decisions' including resuscitation, *see* p. 10.

Advance directives (living wills)

A mentally competent adult may decide how they would like to be treated in the event of them not being able to make these decisions. These 'advance directives' carry the same force as contemporaneous statements made by that individual.

Case 33: Talking about PEG insertion

Candidate information

You are an SHO working on a stroke unit.

Please read the scenario below. You may make notes on the paper provided. When the bell sounds enter the examination room to begin the consultation.

Subject: Mr Colin Banks

Age: 37 years

Re: mother, Mrs Sofia Banks, aged 76 years

A 37-year-old man, Mr Colin Banks, asks to speak to you about his mother who is having a percutaneous (PEG) feeding tube inserted. She had been admitted several weeks previously following a dense stroke. Prior to this episode, the 76-year-old lady had been well, except for hypertension and obesity. There has been some improvement since her admission and she has become alert and gained some use of her right arm and leg, which had been effected by the stroke. She is currently being fed via a nasogastric (NG) tube and has recently had an assessment by a speech and language therapist (SALT), who has deemed her swallowing unsafe. A gastroenterologist has reviewed her and agrees that it is appropriate to insert a PEG feeding tube, although it will be technically challenging because of her obesity. The lady was unable to sign her consent form, but has given a verbal consent. Your objective is to speak to Mr Banks and inform him of what the procedure entails and to answer any questions that he may have.

You have 14 minutes to communicate with the subject followed by one minute for reflection before discussion with the examiners.

Subject information

Mr Colin Banks

Aged 37 years

Re: mother, Mrs Sofia Banks, aged 76 years

This gentleman's mother (Mrs Sofia Banks) was admitted to hospital some weeks ago following a stroke. Prior to this the 76-year-old lady had only suffered with hypertension and obesity. Since her admission, there has been some improvement in her symptoms and in particular Mr Banks is encouraged that she is more alert now and able to move her previously paralysed arm. At present, she is being fed by a nasal feeding tube, but the plan is to insert a gastrostomy feeding tube through the abdominal wall. The nurse looking after his mother told Mr Banks that the procedure can have serious complications, but was unable to give any specific details. Mr Banks has therefore asked to speak to a doctor, and the nurse has summoned the SHO. He specifically intends to ask the doctor about the complications associated with the procedure and the need to have the tube inserted. He is also aware that his mother is not able to sign the consent form and he wants to know if he needs to sign a consent form on her behalf.

Possible prompts

- Mother already has a tube coming out of her nose for feeding. Why does she need another one?
- How is the tube inserted?
- Will it be permanent?
- Are there any problems with the procedure?
- Can she go home with it?
- Do I need to sign her consent form?

Possible interview plan

- Greet the subject and introduce yourself to him.
- Set the agenda. Confirm with him that he has asked to speak with you regarding his mother and the insertion of a feeding tube.

- Ask him what he knows about the procedure and why the tube is being inserted.
- Explain to him that the insertion of a feeding tube through the abdominal wall is a common procedure carried out in patients who are unable to feed themselves. A common reason for this is strokes that can affect the swallowing process, which is the reason his mother is having the tube inserted. Further, explain that the nasogastric tube, which is currently being used, can be very uncomfortable for the patient and hence is not appropriate for long-term use.
- He may then ask you about complications. Briefly explain that the procedure is not without complications (particularly because of the obesity), which include bleeding, perforation and damage of other intra-abdominal organs and infection, but they are rare. It is important to emphasise that you are not a specialist and you could either speak with one to get an exact idea of potential complications or organise a discussion with the specialists.
- He may then ask you whether he needs to sign a consent form on his mother's behalf, as she is unable to.
- Say that would be helpful and that you would arrange an appropriate consent form for his signature, but explain that he is not legally obliged to sign a consent form.
- Ask if he has any other concerns or questions.
- If not, thank him and close the interview.

Ethical issues

Consent issues are extremely important and have previously been covered on p. 2. An important aspect relevant to this case is that of close family members giving consent for medical procedures. When patients are unable to give consent for themselves, it is a common practice to seek consent from family members. However, there is no medicolegal basis for this practice. But it is common sense and good practice to inform close relatives and particularly the next of kin of any medical procedures to be performed.

PEG tubes

These are inserted in patients who are unable to feed for more than a few weeks. For periods less than this, nasogastric feeding tubes can be used. The most common indication for a PEG tube is swallowing difficulties, which may occur after a stroke and with neurological conditions such as motor neurone disease and multiple sclerosis. Other indications include head and neck cancers, and severe motility problems, particularly if the oesophagus is affected (for example in scleroderma). Rarely it may be used in psychiatric patients with eating disorders.

Case 34: My father is MRSA positive

Candidate information

You are the SHO working on a respiratory ward.

Please read the scenario below. You may make notes on the paper provided. When the bell sounds enter the examination room to begin the consultation.

Subject: Mr Eamonn Robertson

Age: 32 years

Re: father, Mr Herbert Robertson, aged 58 years

The sister on the ward asks you to speak to Mr Eamonn Robertson, who is a 32-year-old man. He has been told that his father (Mr Herbert Robertson), who is a patient with COPD, has been moved to a side room on another ward because he was found to be MRSA positive. He is concerned about what impact this will have on his father's health and whether he and his family are at risk, as they have been visiting him. Your task is to discuss his concerns with him.

You have 14 minutes to communicate with the patient's son followed by one minute for reflection before discussion with the examiners.

Subject information

Mr Eamonn Robertson

Aged 32 years

Re: father, Mr Herbert Robertson, aged 58 years

This gentleman's father (Mr Herbert Robertson) was admitted to hospital a week ago with shortness of breath. He is known to suffer with emphysema and was a smoker until last year. He was treated with steroids, antibiotics and nebulisers and is making a gradual recovery. However, Mr Robertson has come to visit his father today only to find out that he has been moved from his normal bed. Upon enquiring, the sister has told him that his father was found to be MRSA positive and was moved to a side room on another ward to contain the infection. Mr Robertson's initial reaction was of anger as he attributed the MRSA (which he knows as the 'super-bug') infection to the general lack of hygiene on the ward. On a previous occasion he had noted that a demented man in another bed had been incontinent of urine and it had taken 20 minutes before a nurse had changed him. On another occasion, he had noticed a doctor examining an unkempt patient and then examining another patient without stopping to wash his hands. He expressed his dissatisfaction to the sister, who has suggested that he should speak with a doctor. He is also worried about the prospect of him and his young children (who regularly visit their grandfather) acquiring MRSA and the potential risks it may pose to them.

Possible prompts

- Where did he catch this bug?
- Is it because of lack of hygiene in the hospital?
- Can it be cured?
- Will my children be affected?
- How do you know they haven't got the bug?
- Does my family need treating?
- Can we continue to visit my father?

Possible interview plan

- Greet the subject and introduce yourself to him.
- Set the agenda. Confirm with him that he has asked to speak with you regarding his father's transfer to another ward.
- Ask him whether he knows why his father was transferred to another ward.
- Confirm that the move was because his father had been found to be MRSA positive and the move to a side room was to contain the spread of this. Explain that MRSA is a bacterium that normally does not cause problems, but is

difficult to treat in vulnerable patients, particularly those with poor immune systems, and hence measures are taken to prevent spread of the infection within hospitals.

- Further explain that he was moved to another ward because of availability of a side room.
- He may suggest that the infection was spread because of poor hygiene. Agree that hygiene certainly plays an important role in the spread of infection, including MRSA, and nowadays hospital policy dictates that all staff observe a strict code of practice for hand washing and the use of alcohol hand rub, which can be more effective than washing.
- If he is not satisfied, allow him to express his concerns regarding hygiene, but reassure him that you will speak with the sister/ward manager and ensure that hand-washing policy is reinforced or adhered to.
- Reassure him that MRSA poses very little risk to him and his family. But if he wants, you can organise for swabs to be taken and if positive, prescribe treatment. Explain to him that because his father is 'barrier nursed' it is important that when they see him they wear aprons and gloves and use the alcohol hand rub provided.
- Ask if he has any other concerns or questions.
- If not, thank him and close the interview.

Healthcare-associated infections

In England approximately 1 in 10 people are admitted to hospital with an infection they developed at home and a further 1 in 10 people admitted to hospitals develop an infection after admission (National Audit Office Report, 2000). Since 2001 hospitals have been required to report certain types of infection to the Department of Health. These include:

- methicillin-resistant *Staphylococcus aureus* (MRSA) septicaemia
- *Clostridium difficile*-associated diarrhoea
- vancomycin-resistant *enterococci* (VRE) septicaemia
- infections following knee and hip replacements.

Over the last decade there has been considerable media interest on this topic and the general consensus has been that poor hygiene was leading to a surge in these infections, increasing patient morbidity and mortality. These concerns have led to the Department of Health's 'Towards cleaner hospitals and lower rates of infection' programme. This programme sets out a strategy to improve the general state of cleanliness within hospitals and thereby reduce the risk of hospital-acquired infections (described as healthcare-associated infections). Key elements to this programme include empowering patients and the public, the matron's charter, independent inspection and learning from the best.

The Department of Health has also suggested that tackling healthcare-associated infection requires commitment from all levels of NHS organisation and cannot be left to clinical staff alone. To this end, directors of infection prevention and control should be employed, who report directly to the trust board. It would be the role of these directors to ensure that infection control is a key part of the NHS organisation.

Case 35: Speak with daughter about mother's death

Candidate information

You are an SHO working on a general medical ward.

Please read the scenario below. You may make notes on the paper provided. When the bell sounds enter the examination room to begin the consultation.

Subject: Mrs Jean Timbury

Age: 51 years

Re: mother, Mrs Eleanor Hodgetts, aged 86 years

Mrs Jean Timbury, a 51-year-old social worker, has arranged to speak with you to discuss the circumstances of her mother's death. The consultant who had looked after her mother had agreed to see her, but unfortunately is away today due to illness and his secretary has asked you to speak to her instead (the team does not have a registrar). Her mother, Mrs Eleanor Hodgetts, was an 86-year-old woman who was known to have long-standing ischemic heart disease and heart failure. Ten days previously she had been admitted with shortness of breath secondary to pulmonary oedema and investigations had shown a likely myocardial infarct. Despite being treated aggressively, including thrombolysis, intravenous diuretics and a nitrate infusion, she deteriorated and died. The medical team had discussed her with the ITU team and it was considered inappropriate to intubate and ventilate. Prior to her death, a registrar had documented Mrs Hodgetts as not for resuscitation, after discussing this with the patient. The death had been expected and had not been referred to the coroner. Your objective is to discuss these issues with Mrs Timbury and to answer any questions she may have.

You have 14 minutes to communicate with the patient's daughter followed by one minute for reflection before discussion with the examiners.

Subject information

Mrs Jean Timbury

Aged 51 years

Re: mother, Mrs Eleanor Hodgetts, aged 86 years

This lady's 86-year-old mother (Mrs Eleanor Hodgetts) was admitted to hospital 10 days ago with shortness of breath and had died the next day. The only significant past medical history is of a heart attack three years previously, which had left her with very mild heart failure and shortness of breath. Mrs Timbury lives in a town 50 miles away and was not able to see her mother during her final illness. She is deeply upset by her sudden death, particularly as she had spoken to her on the day of her admission and she had seemed her normal self. She also feels somewhat guilty because she is an only child and wasn't there at the end. There are lots of questions she would like to have answered and had arranged to speak with the consultant who had looked after her mother. However, Mrs Timbury is annoyed to find out on her arrival at the hospital that the consultant is unable to see her and instead the secretary has arranged a junior doctor to speak with her. Because she has taken the day off work and it has taken her nearly two hours to get to her appointment, she agrees to see the junior doctor. She is particularly anxious to enquire about her mother's management and whether she had been resuscitated. She will be upset to find out that resuscitation had not been attempted and thinks that if it had been she would have been there at the end. However, when the doctor explains the inappropriateness and futility of attempting resuscitation, she will accept this decision.

Possible prompts

- What caused mother's death?
- Could anything have been done to save her?

- One of the nurses told me that she had not been sent for intensive care. Can you tell me why?
- Did you try to resuscitate her?

Possible interview plan

- Greet the subject and introduce yourself to her.
- Set the agenda. Apologise that the consultant is not here to speak with her today because of illness and confirm that she would like to speak about her mother's illness and death.
- Ask her what she knows about her mother's illness. She will tell you that her mother had been well and she had spoken with her on the day she came into hospital. Her understanding is that her mother was brought into hospital with shortness of breath and died shortly afterwards.
- Confirm that her mother had come into hospital with shortness of breath, which was thought to be because of heart failure. Explain that investigations carried out at the time showed that her mother had suffered a heart attack, which had caused the sudden deterioration. Upon admission she had been treated promptly, but despite the best efforts of the medical team had deteriorated and died.
- At this point she may enquire if resuscitation had been attempted.
- Say that it had not. Explain that this is an important decision that the team had made after discussion with the intensive care unit. It was felt that the situation was futile and the lady was unlikely to make a recovery. Gently explain to her that resuscitation in such circumstances generally has a poor outcome and can be an extremely undignified death.
- At this juncture it would be reasonable to pause and allow the subject to express her emotions, and respond to her emotions with empathy and answer any questions she may have.
- Ask if she has any other concerns or questions.
- If not, thank her and close the interview.

Bereavement

Bereavement is a universal human experience and is associated with a high morbidity, where up to one-third of those bereaved may go on to develop a depressive illness. It is well recognised that there are stages in the grief process. But these stages are not often ordered or structured. The basic stages of grief are:

- *initial shock* – there is numbness and shock and the person accepts the reality of the loss
- *pangs of grief* – common emotions experienced here include sadness, vulnerability, anxiety, anger as well as regret, guilt and anger. Insomnia and social withdrawal are also common experiences
- *despair* – the subject feels a loss in their life's direction and is a way of adjusting to a new environment, without a loved one
- *adjustment* – this is the final stage where the bereaved person begins to form new relationships and emotionally relocate the deceased to an important, but not central, place in their life and move on.

This is the normal bereavement process and the bereaved person will go though it and eventually get back to a normal life. The time period over which this happens is variable and depends on multiple factors. Similarly, there are factors that lead to a poor outcome from the process and the bereaved person is more likely to end up clinically depressed and even commit suicide. This is said to be 'complicated grief'. Factors that are likely to lead to complicated grief include:

- close relationship with the deceased
- sudden and unexpected death, particularly of a young person (or worse still, a child), for example following a road traffic accident. This may be even worse if the death had a social stigma attached, for example by suicide, taking a drug overdose or dying of AIDS
- previous mental illness and low self-esteem
- inability to carry out religious/cultural rituals. For instance,

ethnic minority patients often prefer their burial or cremation to take place in the land of their birth with their ancestors. This isn't always practical or possible and the surviving relative may feel immense guilt

- multiple bereavements and life crises
- caring for the deceased for longer than six months
- generally speaking, men fare worse in comparison to women
- lack of social support.

Assessing and treating complicated grief can be complex and is beyond the scope of this present text. Suffice it to say that the therapeutic process encourages the grieving process.

CPR decisions

For a discussion on CPR and other 'end-of-life decisions', including resuscitation, *see* p. 10.

Case 36: Father diagnosed with Huntington's disease

Candidate information

You are a neurology SHO.

Please read the scenario below. You may make notes on the paper provided. When the bell sounds enter the examination room to begin the consultation.

Subject: Mrs Amy Martinez

Age: 29 years

Re: father, Mr Ronald Crichton, aged 59 years

A 26-year-old woman asks to speak to you regarding her father. She normally lives in Canada and is keen to speak to someone as she is flying back home the next day. Her father was admitted several weeks previously with clumsiness and forgetfulness. Although the admitting team felt that he might have had a stroke, your consultant was suspicious of Huntington's disease. Genetic tests were carried out and have confirmed the diagnosis of Huntington's disease. Your task is to explain the diagnosis and its implications to the patient's daughter. She has told one of the nurses that she has recently got married and is keen to start a family.

You have 14 minutes to communicate with the patient's daughter followed by one minute for reflection before discussion with the examiners.

Subject information

Mrs Amy Martinez

Aged 31 years

Re: father, Mr Ronald Crichton, aged 59 years

This lady normally lives in Canada and came to the UK when her 59-year-old father (Mr Ronald Crichton) was admitted to hospital with forgetfulness and clumsiness. The initial diagnosis had been of a stroke, but he was undergoing further tests. Mrs Martinez has recently got married, works as a publishing assistant and normally enjoys good health, working out at the gym three times per week. Both she and her husband are keen to have children. Her flight back to Canada is scheduled for the next day and she has organised to speak to a doctor regarding her father's progress. When she speaks to the doctor, it comes as a shock that her father may have an inheritable condition that has implications for her and her family.

Possible prompts

- Will my father get better?
- Are there any treatments for this condition?
- Will I develop this condition?
- How can I tell if I have the condition?
- Can I be tested now?
- Is there a chance that my children will develop this?

Possible interview plan

- Greet the subject and introduce yourself to her.
- Set the agenda. Confirm that she has asked to speak with you regarding her father's progress.
- Ask her what she has been told about her father's illness thus far. She will tell you that her father is being treated for a suspected stroke, but the doctors have told her that they are carrying out further tests. She does not know what these are for.

- Confirm that there was an initial suspicion that her father had had a stroke. However, your consultant wasn't convinced and was suspicious of a condition called Huntington's disease. Ask her if she has heard of the condition. She will tell you she has not.
- Explain to her that this is a serious condition, which causes a progressive deterioration in both the ability to carry out physical tasks and mental function to the extent that people develop advanced dementia. Say that there is no cure for this condition, but instead management focuses on optimum nursing care and symptom relief.
- Now carefully explain to her that this is an inheritable condition, which has implications for the patient's children, including the lady herself.
- Pause and let her absorb this information and the significance for her.
- Further explain that the risk of developing the disease if one of your parents is affected is 50 per cent and tests are available that will show whether or not an individual is likely to develop the condition. However, testing can only be carried out after formal genetic counselling.
- She may tell you that she is flying to Canada the following day and is worried that she may not be able to seek further advice or genetic counselling. Reassure her that counselling and testing can be carried out in Canada, which can be organised through her own general practitioner and that you would be happy to write a letter for her to take beck to her GP to organise the necessary referral and testing. Remind her that this is an inherited condition and a delay in testing will not make any difference.
- Ask if she has any other concerns or questions.
- If not, thank her and close the interview.

Inherited disease

With scientific advances in molecular biology such as the 'Genome Project', the mechanisms behind inherited disease are becoming clearer and tests are becoming available to test for the presence of genes in a number of conditions. Huntington's chorea or disease (HD) is a condition inherited via an autosomal dominant trait. The responsible gene is present on chromosome 4 and encodes a protein known as *huntingtin*. This protein progressively accumulates within brain cells and damages them by as yet unknown mechanism.

Patients often present with involuntary movements (e.g. piano-playing motion of the fingers or facial grimaces) or rigidity or mental changes, which in the early stages appear as increased irritability, moodiness, or antisocial behaviour. Patients who develop HD by the time they are aged 35 years often become bedridden within 15–20 years and dementia develops as the disease progresses. At present there is no cure for the condition and management is aimed at symptom control and social support. Family history is of paramount importance in making the diagnosis.

Genetic test counselling

Individuals may wish to be tested if:

- they develop symptoms of a heritable condition
- there is a family history of a heritable condition
- they are worried about passing on a heritable condition to their children.

In real life genetic test counselling can be a complex process involving a multidisciplinary team, including for instance, in the case of Huntington's disease, neurologists, geneticists, psychiatrists and counsellors. However, for the purposes of the exam it is important to emphasise that the result of the test has implications for the rest of the patient's own life and their descendants. In addition to personal and family issues, genetic disease or susceptibility may have implications for employment and insurance. Therefore, careful consideration in the handling of this information is very important. Critical issues include:

- *informed consent* – patients must have knowledge of the risks, benefits, effectiveness and alternatives to testing in order to understand the implications of genetic testing. The findings may affect the future employability or insurability of the individual

- *confidentiality and privacy* – the patient must be reassured that access to genetic information will be limited to those authorised to receive it.

The advantage of having the test is to obtain information that will enable the patient to take control of their life. For instance, if it is negative then they can be reassured and lead a normal life and not feel that they have the 'sword of Damocles hanging over their head'*. If on the other hand the test comes back positive, then it will empower the patient to make appropriate lifestyle choices regarding their vocation and starting a family, etc. It is important that you explain the nature of the test, which is usually a blood test, and your follow-up plan. As a general rule, the result should always be given in person and never over the phone or by letter.

* Ancient legend about a man named Damocles who swapped places with a king to enjoy his riches only to find a sword hanging over his head, held by a single horse hair, ready to drop any moment.

Case 37: Stopping ventilation and organ donation

Candidate information

You are the SHO working on a busy ITU.

Please read the scenario below. You may make notes on the paper provided. When the bell sounds enter the examination room to begin the consultation.

Subject: Mr Robert Declan

Age: 63 years

Re: son, Mr Simon Declan, aged 24 years

Simon Declan collapsed at a party. He was subsequently diagnosed with a massive intracranial haemorrhage, possibly secondary to a ruptured berry aneurysm, and required admission to an intensive care unit. He is currently supported on a ventilator and the medical team have conducted tests, which show that he is brainstem dead and that the ventilator should be turned off. You are asked to discuss this with the man's father, who is the next of kin, and also breach the subject of organ donation. There is no other close family. The father, Mr Robert Declan, works as a long-distance lorry driver and has just arrived at the ITU after being informed on his mobile phone that his son had been admitted.

You have 14 minutes to communicate with the patient's father followed by one minute for reflection before discussion with the examiners.

Subject information

Mr Robert Declan

Aged 63 years

Re: son, Simon Declan, aged 24 years

This gentleman works as a long-distance lorry driver and had been away on a job when he received a call on his mobile phone from the police who had simply informed him that his son (Simon Declan, aged 24 years) had been involved in an 'incident' and had been admitted to hospital. Mr Declan divorced his wife many years ago and lives with his son, who is his only child. He arrived at the hospital to find out that his son was in the ITU. Before seeing his son, the nurse has asked him to speak with the SHO. The SHO will inform him that his son collapsed and was brought to hospital, and subsequent tests showed that he had suffered a massive intracranial bleed. The SHO should also explain that tests show that his son is brainstem dead and the ventilator is currently keeping him alive. This news will be devastating, and made worse by the fact that the team intend to turn the ventilator off. In addition, the SHO will discuss the prospect of organ donation and, in particular, seek Mr Declan's consent. Mr Declan will find it all too overwhelming and be unable to give his consent.

Possible prompts

- Will he get better?
- Is it a stroke that he has had?
- But if he is breathing and his heart is beating, how can he be dead?
- Would he be able to hear me if I spoke to him?
- I can't let you cut my boy up.

Possible interview plan

- Greet the subject and introduce yourself to him.
- Set the agenda. Confirm that you have been asked to speak with the gentleman because his son was admitted to the ITU.

- Ask what he knows about his son's admission to hospital. He will tell you that he received a call from the police who said his son had been involved in an 'incident' and admitted to hospital. On arrival at the hospital he was surprised to find out that he had been brought to the intensive care unit.
- Gently explain to him that his son was admitted to hospital after he collapsed at a party and was unconscious when he was brought into hospital and put onto a ventilator (explain what this is). A subsequent scan of his head had shown that he had suffered a large bleed into the brain.
- Pause and let him absorb this information.
- Tell him that further tests were carried out, which suggest that his son is brain dead and not likely to recover from this event; indeed, if the ventilator was stopped he would not be breathing. Further, explain that the situation is futile and that the team plan to switch the ventilator off.
- Pause and let the news sink in (the golden silence).
- Respond to the patient's feelings in an empathetic manner. Answer any immediate questions that he may have.
- If the man is relatively calm, breach the subject of organ donation. Ask if his son had ever mentioned organ donation or had carried an organ donor card and whether the gentleman would consent to the use of his son's organs for transplantation.
- Mr Declan will find this subject highly emotive and will be unable to give consent. It is important that you do not pressurise him into giving consent and it may be appropriate to simply ask him if he would like more time to think about it. If he is adamant that he does not want his son's organs to be transplanted, then reassure him that his wish will be respected.
- Briefly summarise the discussion and ask if he has any further questions.
- Thank him and close the interview.

What are the criteria for brainstem death and how is it established?

Brainstem death can be established when the following brain-stem reflexes are absent:

- no pupillary response to light
- absent corneal reflex
- no motor response within cranial nerve distribution
- absent gag reflex
- absent cough reflex
- absent vestibulo-ocular reflex.

Persistant aponea must be confirmed as follows:

- the patient must be pre-oxygenated with 100 per cent oxygen for 10 minutes and $PaCO_2$ allowed to rise above 5.0 kPa
- disconnect the patient from the ventilator
- during the test while maintaining adequate oxygenation, allow $PaCO_2$ to climb above 6.65 kPa and confirm that there is no spontaneous respiration
- reconnect the ventilator.

Two experienced physicians must carry out these tests, at least one of whom must be a consultant and neither should be part of a transplant team. The tests have to be carried out on two separate occasions.

What criteria need to be excluded before brainstem death can be diagnosed?

Neurological examination to determine whether a patient is brain dead can proceed only if the following prerequisites are met: the ruling out of complicated medical conditions that may confound the clinical assessment, particularly severe electrolyte, acid-base, or endocrine disturbances; the absence of severe hypothermia, defined as a core temperature of 32°C or lower; hypotension; and the absence of evidence of drug intoxication, poisoning, or neuromuscular blocking agents.

What do you understand by the terms 'locked-in syndrome' and 'persistent vegetative state'?

The *locked-in syndrome* is a state of unresponsiveness, due to massive brainstem infarction. The patient has a functioning cerebral cortex, and is thus aware, but cannot move or communicate except by vertical eye movement. The *persistent vegetative state*, a sequel of, for example, widespread cortical damage after head injury, implies loss of sentient behaviour. The patient perceives little or nothing but lies apparently awake, breathing spontaneously.

Do you think there should be a mandatory organ-donor system?

The advantage of a 'mandatory organ-donor system' is that it would allow viable organs to be salvaged from dead patients without the requirement for consent. This would solve the national shortage of organs. The problem with this is that it violates patient's autonomy and is against the basic principles of medical ethics.

Are you aware of any legislation related to organ donation?

In previous years two key laws governed organ donation and transplantation:

1 The Human Tissue Act 1961, and
2 The Human Organ Transplants Act 1989.

However, following recent scandals such as that at Bristol Royal Infirmary and Alder Hay, where human tissue was removed without consent, the government reviewed and repealed these Acts in favour of the Human Tissue Act 2004. Under this Act *consent* is the fundamental principle underpinning the lawful use of, and retention of, organs, body parts and tissue. The Act also established the *Human Tissue Authority* to advise on and oversee compliance with the Act. 'Appropriate consent' is required for lawful storage or use of human tissue, which includes tissue obtained for transplant purposes. Appropriate consent can be obtained as follows:

- from a living competent adult, or competent child willing to make a decision
- from a person with parental responsibility for an incompetent child
- for a deceased person (as in this case), where consent has not been obtained from the patient during their life, consent may be obtained from a *qualifying relative*. A qualifying relative may be any of the following:
  - spouse or partner
  - parent or child
  - brother or sister
  - grandparent or grandchild
  - child of a brother or sister
  - stepfather or stepmother
  - half-brother or half-sister
  - friend of long standing.

What does the term 'presumed consent' mean to you?

There is a chronic shortage of organs for transplantation. This is despite the fact that most people when polled say that they would be happy for their organs to be used after their death. One potential solution is to institute a law where there is 'presumed consent' for organs to be used after their death, unless the patient has specifically stated to the contrary. This is not a new idea and indeed France has had such a policy since 1976. Other European countries, including Austria, Belgium, Denmark, Finland, Italy, Norway and Spain, have laws that give physicians the right to presume that a deceased person is an organ donor unless they have signed a written directive, or have registered in a computer data bank, indicating that they do not wish to do so.

Reference

Wijdicks EFM (2001) The diagnosis of brain death. *NEJM.* **344**: 1215–21.

Case 38: Transplant 1 – The living donor

Candidate information

You are the SHO working on a renal transplant unit.

Please read the scenario below. You may make notes on the paper provided. When the bell sounds enter the examination room to begin the consultation.

Subject: Mrs Kathleen Hoole

Age: 58 years

Re: daughter, Miss Neve Hoole, aged 19 years

This lady's daughter (Neve Hoole) has been a patient under regular follow-up for four years and has now developed end-stage renal disease, requiring dialysis three times per week. Her renal disease is thought to be secondary to chronic glomerulonephritis. Although she is on a waiting list for a cadaveric transplant, it has been previously explained to the patient and her family that there was no guarantee that she would get a suitable kidney and people can be waiting for a transplant for years before one is found. The possibility of getting a kidney from a living donor has been mentioned, but not discussed. The patient's mother, Mrs Kathleen Hoole, has come to the clinic today to explore this option further. Your consultant has asked you to have a frank discussion with the mother about living/related donation of a kidney, while he sees the patient and continues with the very busy clinic. Your task is to give Mrs Hoole an overview, including any pros and cons, of acting as a living donor and to answer any questions that she may have.

You have 14 minutes to communicate with the patient's mother followed by one minute for reflection before discussion with the examiners.

Subject information

Mrs Kathleen Hoole

Aged 58 years

Re: daughter, Miss Neve Hoole, aged 19 years

This lady's daughter was diagnosed with renal failure secondary to chronic glomerulonephritis four years ago and is now on haemodyalisis three times per week. She has been placed on a waiting list for a renal transplant, but the doctor looking after her has previously said that it was impossible to predict how long she would have to wait before a kidney became available, and often people were waiting for years and indeed many people never receive a transplant. He had also mentioned the possibility of relatives donating one of their kidneys, but because of constraints of time had been unable to elaborate on this. Mrs Hoole is very worried about her daughter and her future and thinks that a renal transplant is the only hope for a normal quality of life for her. Because of this, she is seriously considering donating one of her kidneys to her daughter, but needs more information. Today she has accompanied her daughter to a follow-up appointment at the renal unit to discuss this option further. The consultant at the clinic has arranged for her to have a discussion with one of the junior doctors.

Possible prompts

- I would like to discuss my daughter's kidney disease.
- We have been waiting for a long time. What is the prospect of her getting a kidney transplant?
- I am seriously considering the possibility of giving one of my kidneys to her. Can you give me some information on this?
- If I gave one of my kidneys, would I end up on dialysis?
- Is it a safe procedure?
- How long would I have to take off work to donate a kidney?
- What happens next?

The interview

- Introduce yourself to the subject.
- Confirm that she is here to discuss renal transplantation and possibly acting as a donor, and enquire about any specific questions that she may have.
- Explore her motivation to act as a living donor.
- Explain, in non-medical jargon what a renal transplant involves and why there is a need for living donors. Discuss potential complications, including the prospect of the transplant failing to function. However, medical data show that 95 per cent of transplants are functioning at one year and this continues to improve. It is important that the donor realises that the assessment process (as outlined below) is a long one and that the surgery involves a major operation that can result in life-threatening complications and at the very least, pain.
- It is easy to be negative, but perhaps it is also worth bringing up the positive aspects of becoming a donor, such as being able to give a loved one a near-normal quality of life.
- Don't forget to mention the practical implications for the donor, such as having to spend a week in hospital and a further 8–12 weeks off work. Also, they may need to speak to their insurers to see what implications there are for any life cover, etc.
- Confirm and summarise information at each step.
- Offer to answer any further questions.
- Give a follow-up plan to the lady, such as giving her contact details of the transplant coordinator, and a detailed leaflet giving her more information to be read at leisure.
- Thank the subject and close.

Donor assessment

This is a long drawn-out process (and rightly so!) where the donor is carefully evaluated in terms of medical and psychological well being before a transplant can be carried out. The essential process is as follows:

1   Review by nephrologists, where information and literature are supplied. An opportunity may be given to visit the transplant unit. The donor's blood group must be shown to be compatible with the recipient. Discussion should include the sensitive nature of the tests to be performed and their potential implications. For example, HIV and hepatitis B and C have to be tested for, which has long-term implications for the donor. Moreover, the tests may reveal that individuals are not biologically related!

2   The full biochemical and haematological profile of the potential donor is obtained as well as chest X-ray, ECG and urinanalysis. A detailed virology screen and tissue typing tests are also carried out.

3   If the results from the above tests are acceptable then detailed radiological testing of the kidneys is carried out. This should included a renal ultrasound scan as well as nuclear medicine scans (GFR as well as MAG3 or DTPA scans).

4   At this stage the donor should be formally referred to a transplant surgeon by the recipient's nephrologist, with the involvement of a transplant coordinator. The surgeon will then review the donor and request a renal arteriogram, which can be analysed with the aid of a radiologist. At this stage the donor may be reviewed by an independent professional such as another nephrologist or a counsellor.

5   If the whole of this process is carried out satisfactorily, only then can it proceed to a renal transplant.

The whole process may take 3–6 months to complete.

Ethical and legal issues

There are many ethical issues surrounding live organ donation, of which perhaps the most significant is the right to remove an organ from a healthy individual and the potential risks that carries. Does the principle of 'non-maleficence' (doing no harm) to the donor outweigh the 'beneficence' (doing good) for the recipient? There are many differing opinions surrounding this argument. There is a real concern regarding possible pressures or even coercion placed upon donors by families, recipients, or even the transplant teams. This is particularly so because of the altruistic nature of acting as a living donor, be it a related donor (parent, sibling, etc.) or an unrelated donor (such as spouse or close friend). But perhaps true altruism only occurs when there is no emotional attachment to the patient.

Perhaps the most controversial issue surrounding live organ donation is the sale of organs – so-called 'trafficking'. It is well recognised that there is an underground industry in exploiting poor and vulnerable people across the globe for this purpose. Indeed, even in Britain, trafficking of organs by a surgeon led to the formation of the Human Organ Transplants Act in 1989. This clearly states that organs cannot be exchanged for money. The World Health Organization (WHO) (1991) says that a 'Rational argument can be made to the effect that shortage has led to the rise of commercial traffic in human organs, particularly from donors who are unrelated to recipients . . .'. There is also an argument that with the severe shortage of donor organs are we morally justified in denying patients the option of buying organs, if others are willing to sell their organs (Bartucci, 1990).

References

Bartucci MR (1990) ANNAgrams Q:A. *ANNA J.* **17**(4): 325.

World Health Organization (1991) Guiding principles on human organ transplantation. *The Lancet.* **337**: 1470–1.

Case 39: Transplant 2 – The paracetamol overdose

Candidate information

You are the RMO on-call.

Please read the scenario below. You may make notes on the paper provided. When the bell sounds enter the examination room to begin the consultation.

Subject: Mr Todd Panos

Age: 49 years

Re: daughter, Miss Natasha Panos, aged 18 years

You had admitted this 18-year-old girl earlier in the day. Two days ago, she had taken 50 paracetamol tablets after learning that she had failed her 'A' level exams and would not be going to university. She had been admitted today with nausea, vomiting and jaundice. Blood tests had confirmed a raised bilirubin and abnormal urea and electrolytes. Her clotting was also found to be deranged with a raised prothrombin time. N-acetyl cystine (Parvolex) had been promptly commenced and you had chosen to discuss the case with the registrar on call for the liver unit. She had been extremely concerned about this girl's failing liver and after discussing the case with her consultant, has agreed to transfer her to the liver unit as she almost certainly will require a liver transplant. Natasha's father, Mr Todd Panos, has asked to speak to you about his daughter's progress. He is unaware of the paracetamol overdose, and Natasha has asked you not to discuss this with him, but she is happy for you to relay other information to him, including the prospect of a liver transplant. Your objective is to do this.

You have 14 minutes to communicate with the patient's father followed by one minute for reflection before discussion with the examiners.

Subject information

Mr Todd Panos

Aged 49 years

Re: daughter, Miss Natasha Panos, aged 18 years

This man had been informed at work that his daughter had become 'poorly', and had required hospital admission. Upon arrival at the hospital he was surprised to find her looking very unwell with vomiting, and she appeared confused and drowsy, to the point where she barely recognised him. He also noticed that she appeared yellow. Normally his daughter was an intelligent and vibrant girl, but had recently been a little down after doing badly with her 'A' level exams. He normally lives with his wife, who is away on business, and Natasha, his younger daughter. His other daughter is away at university. He loves his children very much and is concerned about this sudden illness. The nurse caring for Natasha is unable to clarify the cause and degree of illness, except that it is related to her liver and organised for him to have a discussion with the admitting doctor, who he is about to meet. He is particularly keen to find out about the cause for the sudden deterioration and will ask the question directly.

Possible prompts

- I wanted to talk to someone about my daughter. Can you tell me how she is doing?
- I understand it's something to do with her liver. Can you tell me more?
- What caused this problem with her liver?
- I noticed that she was quite drowsy. Is this likely to be related?
- When will she get better and go home?
- A liver transplant sounds very serious. Is it a risky procedure?

- When will she have her liver transplanted?

Possible interview plan

- Greet and introduce yourself to the subject.
- Confirm that he is the father of the patient and would like to discuss the progress of his daughter.
- Ask what he knows of her current condition.
- If he is unaware of the severity of his daughter's condition, then explain the nature of and severity of her illness, i.e. acute onset liver failure, without going into the details of the suspected aetiology.
- However, it may become difficult if he asks the question directly. You could either say that you are not able to give him an answer, as the information is confidential, or instead say that it is under investigation.
- Explain that the patient has been discussed with the liver specialists who plan to take over her care. But it is likely to proceed to a liver transplant. You do not need to know the details of the operation, except that it carries a high morbidity and mortality, and depends upon finding a suitable donor. The team working at the liver unit would clarify the details of the operation.
- Answer any other questions without breaching the patient's confidentiality.
- Close the discussion.

Ethical issues

Any information related to a patient is *confidential* and cannot be divulged to third parties except under certain circumstances (*see* p. 7). Often a doctor has to use their discretion and judgement as to who can have what information, and in real life we have to have frank discussions with close relatives and explain to them that their loved one is sick and may die. However, if the patient has specifically stated that information is to be kept confidential then this wish has to be respected.

The ethical issues surrounding live liver donation are even more complex than renal transplantation (refer to the previous case). This is particularly because partial-liver donation carries a much higher morbidity (Surman, 2002) in comparison to live renal donation. In addition, liver failure is often self-inflicted, for example alcohol abuse and paracetamol overdose.

Reference

Surman OS (2002) The ethics of partial-liver donation. *NEJM.* **346**: 1038.

Case 40: Parkinson's disease

Candidate information

You are the SHO on a care of the elderly ward.

Please read the scenario below. You may make notes on the paper provided. When the bell sounds enter the examination room to begin the consultation.

Subject: Mrs Sheila Hopkins

Age: 69 years

Re: husband, Mr Peter Hopkins, aged 73 years

You are asked to speak to Mrs Sheila Hopkins, whose husband is a patient under your care. He is a 73-year-old man, who had originally presented with a lobar pneumonia. Upon recovery, he was diagnosed with Parkinson's disease, by a very experienced consultant, and commenced on therapy with Sinemet. Your objective is to explain the diagnosis, the management and the likely prognosis.

You have 14 minutes to communicate with the patient's wife followed by one minute for reflection before discussion with the examiners.

Subject information

Mrs Sheila Hopkins

Aged 69 years

Re: husband, Mr Peter Hopkins, aged 73 years

This lady's husband, Mr Peter Hopkins, was admitted to hospital with pneumonia, and after treatment has made a good recovery. However, it was noted that he had a tremor and an experienced geriatrician has confidently made the diagnosis of Parkinson's disease and has initiated treatment with Sinamet. This tremor has been present for some time now and Mr Hopkins' mobility has also been worsening. Previously he has been fit and well and enjoyed an active lifestyle. Mrs Hopkins has found her husband's increasing disability a great strain, as she has had to help him with many of his activities of daily living. They live alone, receive no additional help and have one son, but he lives in Australia. She is concerned about her husband's diagnosis, particularly as she has a brother who has Alzheimer's disease and is very confused. She understands Parkinson's disease to be a similar condition, which causes progressive confusion and disability, and is worried about her abilities to cope. She has asked to speak to a doctor and the SHO is about to discuss her husband's diagnosis and answer any questions she may have.

Possible prompts

- I have a brother with Alzheimer's disease, who has become very confused. Is my husband likely to go the same way?
- Will he lose power in his arms and legs?
- Can he die from this?
- Is there any effective treatment?
- We live alone – our only son lives in Australia. How will we cope?

Possible interview plan

- Greet and introduce yourself to the subject.
- Confirm that she is here to discuss her husband's diagnosis.
- Explore her understanding of the diagnosis and explore any specific issues that she may have.
- Confirm or refute any preconceptions and explain the nature of the diagnosis and its management. In particular, reassure her that there is good therapy available for Parkinson's disease and patients often make a dramatic improvement with their mobility.
- Explore concerns regarding social support and reassure her that her husband will be referred to an occupational therapist for assessment. The occupational therapist may visit their home and, if appropriate, will refer to a social worker to organise support services.

- Answer any remaining questions.
- Close the interview.

Parkinson's syndrome

The syndrome essentially consists of a triad of tremor, rigidity and bradykinesia. Classically the rigidity at the elbow joint is described as 'clasp-knife', and when combined with the tremor at the wrist, is said to be 'cog-wheel'. Parkinson's disease per se is due to degeneration of dopiminergic neurones in the substantia nigra. Other causes of the Parkinsonian syndrome include:

- drugs: particularly neuroleptics (e.g. stemetil, metoclopramide)
- brain damage, for example from carbon monoxide poisoning, anoxia, tumours, etc.
- arteriosclerosis
- rarely postencephalitic (c.f. encephalitis lethargica pandemic 1916–1928)
- neurosyphylis
- Wilson's disease
- Parkinson plus syndromes, see below.

Parkinson plus syndromes are multisystem disorders with some features of Parkinson's disease. The two typically described are:

1 multisystem atrophy (formerly Shy-Drager syndrome): a combination of Parkinsonism with orthostatic hypotension, atonic bladder, impotence and urinary incontinenece
2 supranuclear gaze palsy (Steel-Richardson-Olszewski syndrome): there is absent vertical gaze, corrected by moving the head itself. This is associated with axial rigidity and a tendency to fall backwards. Often there is associated dementia.

Benign essential tremor

Patients are often given a presumptive diagnosis of Parkinson's disease, which causes unnecessary distress. The tremor tends to be exacerbated by stress and helped by alcohol (drinking should not be encouraged however!). Occasionally patients find beta-blockers and benzodiazepines useful.

Case 41: Requesting a postmortem

Candidate information

You are an SHO on an infectious diseases ward.

Please read the scenario below. You may make notes on the paper provided. When the bell sounds enter the examination room to begin the consultation.

Subject: Mrs Alice O'Mally

Age: 75 years

Re: husband, Mr Callum O' Mally, aged 73 years

This man has been under the care of your team for about a month. He was originally admitted with pyrexia and lethargy. Multiple investigations had failed to show any evidence of sepsis, although the team had elected to treat him blindly with broad-spectrum antibiotics. Other investigations had also been unrewarding, apart from a CT scan of the abdomen, which had demonstrated enlarged lymph nodes around the coeliac axis, which were suspicious of lymphoma. Despite the best efforts of the team, Mr O'Mally is deteriorating and expected to die. Throughout the illness his wife, Mrs Alice O'Mally, has been visiting on a daily basis and you have spoken with her on a number of occasions, including recently when you had explained that his prognosis was extremely poor and that the team had decided that he should not be resuscitated in the event of a cardiac arrest. Now he has Cheyne-Stoke respiration and is expected to die soon. Because a firm diagnosis has never been established, the consultant has asked you to speak to his wife with a view to obtaining her consent for a postmortem examination. You arrange a discussion with Mrs O'Mally in a side room. Your objective is to have a frank discussion with the lady and try to obtain her consent for a postmortem.

You have 14 minutes to communicate with the patient's wife followed by one minute for reflection before discussion with the examiners.

Subject information

Mrs Alice O'Mally

Aged 75 years

Re: husband, Mr Callum O' Mally, aged 73 years

Mr O'Mally was admitted to hospital about a month ago with a pyrexia and lethargy. The team looking after him suspected an infection and carried out multiple investigations to find the source. This proved unsuccessful, but they chose to treat with antibiotics anyway. A CT scan of the abdomen had shown enlarged lymph nodes around the aorta, but there was no easy way to biopsy these. The SHO (the candidate) looking after her husband has had a few discussions with Mrs O'Mally over the course of the month to keep her informed of his progress. During their last discussion she was depressed to hear that the team considered his prognosis futile and had declared him not for resuscitation in the event of a cardiac arrest. Mrs O'Mally is a deeply religious woman and has accepted her husband's imminent death and simply wants him now to die with dignity and in peace. However, as she sits at her husband's bedside, she is surprised that the SHO has asked to speak with her again. During the course of their discussion she is horrified to hear that he is proposing a postmortem examination, which will involve a pathologist opening him up, and possibly retaining his organs. Her instincts tell her that he should be buried whole. Although she finds the idea of a postmortem abhorrent, during the course of their discussion she understands the rationale for conducting the procedure and reluctantly agrees to it being carried out, but on the proviso that no organs are removed prior to his burial.

Possible prompts

- Yes I realise he is extremely poorly and will die soon.
- What exactly does a postmortem examination involve?

- Does that mean they will cut him up?
- Would they keep his organs? I couldn't cope with him not being buried whole.
- Will this postmortem definitely give you the cause for his illness?
- I understand the importance of this test and agree to it being carried out, but no organs should be removed under any circumstances.

Possible interview plan

- Greet the subject and thank her for having this discussion with you.
- Explain that your consultant has asked you to speak with her regarding her husband's illness and the team not being able to get a firm diagnosis. Reiterate the fact that over the course of the month multiple investigations have been carried out, which have not yielded the diagnosis but a CT scan of the abdomen had shown evidence of enlarged nodes, which could be a cancer.
- Allow her to respond during the course of this discussion. She may say that she understands all this, but what is the point of the discussion today.
- Go on to explain that the consultant has proposed a postmortem investigation to gain further insight into his final illness.
- Pause and allow her to reflect on this information and respond. She is likely to be upset and very much against the idea of him undergoing a postmortem and argue that it's not going to make any difference to him after his death.
- Explain the rationale for conducting a postmortem, namely that it's unsatisfactory for the team not to have made a diagnosis and to be certain that he was not denied any treatment that could have potentially saved his life. Moreover, the results could influence our practice if placed in a similar situation in the future and could have bearing upon the treatments of other patients. Also, families often feel it easier to deal with bereavement if the cause is identified and

they have the knowledge that nothing else could have been done to alter the course of the illness.

- Allow her to respond. She is likely to be concerned about the disfiguring aspect of the examination and the possibility that organs may be retained. She will be adamant that she wants him to be buried whole and not to have any organs retained.
- You should reassure her that an experienced pathologist will carry out the procedure and generally there are no visible wounds at the funeral. It would be inappropriate to go into the gory details unless she specifically requests the information. Also, you should explain that occasionally organs need to be retained to aid diagnosis and for research purposes, but if she does not agree, then this will not be done. Explain that the postmortem is generally done within a few days of the death and need not delay the funeral.
- If she still declines for the postmortem to go ahead, respect her wishes and reassure her that it will not be carried out. If, on the other hand, she agrees to the postmortem then suggest that you will obtain a consent form and get her consent before the procedure. You will also organise a follow-up appointment with the consultant to discuss the results of the postmortem.
- Close the interview.

The postmortem examination

The postmortem is a detailed examination carried out by a pathologist, looking for evidence of a disease process. This starts off as an external inspection before proceeding to the internal examination. Incisions are kept to a minimum, depending on which organs are to be examined. During a *full* examination, all the organs of the body are removed and inspected before returning them to the body. If a *limited* examination is to be conducted then certain organs may not be inspected, depending upon the constraints of the obtained consent. Organs may be kept for a number of reasons, which include:

- where further analysis is deemed necessary to determine cause of death. This may for instance occur if the

pathologist wishes to seek the advice of a second pathologist or tests are being carried out, which take time to process
- for research purposes
- for education and training, including placement in a medical museum.

Families and postmortems: a code of practice

Following the Alder Hay and Bristol scandals in recent years, there has been much public debate on postmortem examinations and particularly tissue/organ retention. New legislation in this area is pending, but as an interim measure, 'Families and post mortems: a code of practice' has been published (available on the DoH website – www.dh.gov.uk/assetRoot/04/05/43/12/04054312.pdf). This website also shows consent forms that can be used to obtain consent from next of kin. After looking at the consent forms it should be very obvious whether permission is granted for a full or limited examination and whether permission has been given for organ retention.

Important passages from this code of practice are shown here:

Post mortem examination is crucially important in informing relatives, clinicians and legal authorities on the cause of death, and in telling bereaved families (who wish to know) about the possibility of acquired and genetic diseases which might need care and treatment. More widely, it is important in improving clinical care, maintaining clinical standards, increasing our understanding of disease, preventing the spread of infectious diseases, and in supporting clinical research and training. Respectful and sensitive communication with bereaved families is essential, both to help them take important decisions at a difficult time, and to ensure continuing improvements in future care.

In any setting (NHS, academic or other), human tissue or organs may only be removed, retained, or used if there is a proper accountability framework in place which ensures that valid authority is obtained. Before commencing the procedure, the pathologist is responsible for checking that the post mortem examination and any retention or use have been properly authorised, either through the completion of a consent form which must at least meet the standards required by this document, or by the coroner.

A hospital, or consented, post mortem examination is carried out at the request of the family or the hospital to gain a fuller understanding of the deceased's illness or the cause of death, and to enhance future medical care. During the post mortem examination tissue or whole organs (e.g. the heart) may be preserved for diagnosis, for therapeutic purposes, for future medical education (including assuring the quality of clinical care through audit) or for research. If this happens, it must be in accordance with the provisions of the Human Tissue Act 1961. The valid consent of the family or those close to the deceased person must be given before the post mortem is undertaken to ensure proper compliance with the Act (unless the person who has died has already made a request).

. . . consent MUST be obtained for a hospital post mortem, and for the retention and use of organs and tissue in research or education following either a hospital or coroner's post mortem. The 1961 Act used the term 'spouse' or 'surviving relative' to define those to be consulted. Contemporary families may often involve more complex relationships than the traditional spouse or blood relatives – for example, co-habitation without marriage, including with a same-sex partner, or a longstanding relationship without co-habitation. Professionals involved in talking with families and others about consent need to be aware that identifying the most appropriate person to give consent may not be straightforward and staff must be careful not to make assumptions. Careful judgment is needed in each individual case. All competent adult patients are asked to nominate their next-of-kin formally on admission to hospital. Wherever possible, trusts should make clear to patients the reasons for this nomination, and its potential significance (i.e. that this is not simply a contact number). They ought also to make clear that the person nominated as next-of-kin does not necessarily need to be a blood relative or spouse, and may be a same-sex partner, or even a close friend. The last may be particularly appropriate where the individual does not have a close relationship with any family members. Where an individual does nominate such a person, he or she must consider the nominated person's willingness to act in the event of the individual's incapacity or death. It may be helpful for all concerned for NHS trusts to provide such information and advice clearly and routinely in a short information leaflet.

There is no legal obligation to obtain consent from the family if, in accordance with Section 1(1) of the Human Tissue Act 1961, the deceased has left clear instructions, preferably in writing, that his or her body or tissues should be used for transplantation, medical education or research. However, hospitals might prefer nevertheless to discuss this with the family and consider not going ahead with a post mortem or other procedure in the face of refusal or strong opposition from them, in order to avoid any upsetting conflict at a difficult time, or exacerbating the sense of loss. In any case, they will need to discuss the timing of the funeral, and how this might be affected by a post mortem examination.

In some religions (including the Jewish, Muslim and Hindu faiths), it is important that a funeral should take place as soon as possible, usually within 24 hours. In such cases, every effort should be made to carry out a post mortem examination within that period (if one is required). If this is not likely to be practicable, or if organs cannot be returned within that period, this should be explained to relatives. The family will need the help of hospital staff to get the necessary certification completed urgently before the funeral. In the case of a coroner's post mortem, relatives do not have the option of refusing it, but may want to discuss with the coroner's staff the practical or spiritual implications of any delay.

Case 42: Seeking consent from a relative

Candidate information

You are the SHO on call for medicine.

Please read the scenario below. You may make notes on the paper provided. When the bell sounds enter the examination room to begin the consultation.

Subject: Mr Colin Steel

Age: 48 years

Re: sister, Miss Lucy Steel, aged 52 years

Miss Lucy Steel is a 52-year-old patient with Down's syndrome. She was admitted to hospital with a presumed urinary tract infection, which was treated with antibiotics. However, routine blood tests showed a pancytopenia, suggestive of bone marrow failure. A haematologist who suspects malignant pathology infiltrating the bone marrow has reviewed her. He has therefore recommended a bone marrow biopsy. The problem is that the lady has cognitive impairment and possible early dementia, and is unable to consent to the procedure. Hence your registrar has asked you to call in the patient's documented next of kin, her brother Mr Colin Steel, in an attempt to obtain his consent for the procedure. Mr Steel has arrived in the ward and your task is to discuss the pros and cons of the procedure and obtain his consent. A significant issue is that the procedure will be done under heavy sedation and perhaps even under a general anaesthetic.

You have 14 minutes to communicate with the patient's brother followed by one minute for reflection before discussion with the examiners.

Subject information

Mr Colin Steel

Aged 48 years

Re: sister, Miss Lucy Steel, aged 52 years

Miss Lucy Steel is a 52-year-old patient with Down's syndrome, who normally resides in a care home, where she is very happy. She has cognitive impairment, which is progressively deteriorating and it is suspected that she has early dementia. This admission to hospital was arranged by her GP after a deterioration that was thought to be secondary to a urinary tract infection. She was treated with antibiotics and is slowly recovering. However, routine blood tests have shown a pancytopenia, which the team plan to investigate with a bone marrow biopsy after consulting a haematologist. Because of her poor insight, Lucy is unable to give consent to the procedure and hence the team have called her brother Colin in for a discussion. He is four years her junior and the only living relative. Despite her disability, Colin has always been fond of his sister and is keen to make the right decision on her behalf. The SHO looking after her (the candidate) will have a detailed discussion with Colin about his sister's illness. In particular, he should explain the procedure (the bone marrow biopsy) and that it will be done either under heavy sedation or even a general anaesthetic, and the risks this entails. He should go on to explain that Colin is not under any obligation to give consent on his sister's behalf and indeed, any intervention is decided by the consultant looking after her, who acts in her best interest. Colin will understand all this and agree that all decisions should be left to the medical team, but he is keen to emphasise that his sister should not suffer unduly.

Possible prompts

- I understand Lucy has a waterworks infection, which is getting better.
- What does this bone marrow biopsy involve?
- Will it be painful for her?

- Are there any risks?
- Will it show the problem?
- Do I have to sign the form?
- Of course I want the best for Lucy and I leave her care in the doctor's hands.
- I really don't want her to suffer anymore.

Possible interview plan

- Greet the subject and thank him for having this discussion with you.
- Establish that he is Lucy Steel's next of kin.
- Enquire into his current understanding of her illness and investigation plan.
- Confirm the aspects of his response with which you agree and correct any misconceptions. Expand on important issues in detail, particularly the need to carry out a bone marrow biopsy following a specialist review, as you suspect that there is bone marrow failure.
- Explain that a bone marrow biopsy is an invasive procedure that can be painful and requires a cooperative patient. Hence, because of his sister's lack of insight into her illness and the procedure, it is probably best carried out with heavy sedation or general anaesthesia, and explain the risks this entails. Explain the alternatives (obtaining a fine needle aspirate or not doing an investigation of any kind) and their pros and cons. Remember this discussion could get very drawn out and the skill is to do it within the 14-minute time-frame.
- Confirm his understanding.
- Go on to explain that legally only competent adults are allowed to give consent for themselves. Where the patient lacks capacity, the consultant looking after the patient must make decisions on her behalf, but as a general rule we like to discuss any major treatment issues with the patient's family.
- Again confirm understanding.
- If the subject agrees to the proposed treatment of his relative, then thank him and offer to answer any further

questions. If he has strong objections then reiterate the point that it is a medical decision made in the patient's best interest, but that you can organise a further appointment with the consultant looking after the patient to discuss the issues further.

- Close the interview.

Ethical issues

The key ethical issue surrounding this case is of *consent* (*see* p. 2). As previously stated, an adult and competent patient can make decisions about their treatment and refuse treatment even if it is potentially life-saving. However, when the patient lacks capacity, decisions about their management must be made 'in their best interest' by the doctor in charge of their care, under the auspices of common law. However, it is always a good idea and indeed good practice to maintain good communication with the family and particularly the next of kin. It is crucial to respect the patient's *confidentiality* and *dignity*, even if the patient is incapacitated. Any information disclosed must be appropriate to the discussion and never unnecessary.

Case 43: The Jehovah's Witness

Candidate information

You are the SHO on call for medicine.

Please read the scenario below. You may make notes on the paper provided. When the bell sounds enter the examination room to begin the consultation.

Subject: Mrs Linda Harbottle

Age: 51 years

Re: son, Brian Harbottle, aged 27 years

You have been asked to speak with Mrs Linda Harbottle, who is the mother of Mr Brian Harbottle. Brian is a 27-year-old man who is a strict Jehovah's Witness, although his parents are atheists. He normally works as a motorcycle courier, and was admitted earlier in the day following an accident that had resulted in a significant bleed from his leg; there was no injury to the bone. He was treated by the casualty staff and had required stitches. The bleed has stopped now and no further surgical intervention is needed. However, he was referred to the medical team as his haemaglobin was estimated at 5.6 g/dl. A blood transfusion was planned, but after a lengthy discussion with the consultant looking after him this was refused, and now he is simply being treated with ferrous sulphate and observation. His mother is concerned that without a blood transfusion he may die. Your objective is to discuss the management of Brian Harbottle (who has consented to this discussion) with his mother and answer any questions that she may have.

You have 14 minutes to communicate with the patient's mother followed by one minute for reflection before discussion with the examiners.

Subject information

Mrs Linda Harbottle

Aged 51 years

Re: son, Mr Brian Harbottle, aged 27 years

This lady's son was involved in a motorcycle accident that resulted in a significant bleed from his leg. He required stitches to his leg and the bleeding has stopped. However, his haemaglobin was found to be 5.6 g/dl and hence he has been admitted to hospital. The admitting team suggested a blood transfusion, but Brian refused as he is a strict Jehovah's Witness and accepting blood products is against his faith. Instead, he has elected to take iron tablets and be observed in hospital for a short period. His mother is very concerned, especially as she was told in casualty that a man normally has haemoglobin above 13 g/dl. She is also angry with the medical team for not going against her son's wishes and transfusing him anyway by way of applying a section. She knows about sections as her sister who suffers with schizophrenia once underwent one after she became delirious. Mrs Harbottle has little time for her son's faith and feels that he has been brainwashed by religious fanatics. She herself is an atheist. She has organised an appointment with one of the doctors looking after her son to find out more about his medical problems and to suggest that they should transfuse him against his wishes.

Possible prompts

- I don't understand what haemoglobin of 5.6 means. Is that very low?
- Is this life-threatening? Can he die?
- Why can't you force him to have a blood transfusion, if it is in his best interest?
- I thought doctors could section patients. Is that not the case?
- How long will these iron tablets take to work?
- What if his leg starts to bleed again?

Possible interview plan

- Greet and introduce yourself to the subject.
- Enquire about Mrs Harbottle's understanding of her son's medical condition and her specific concerns. She will tell you that he is anaemic, following his bleed and in her opinion requires a blood transfusion.
- Agree that haemaglobin of 5.6 g/dl is low, but reassure her that people with even worse anaemia have made a full recovery.
- Explain to her that a blood transfusion cannot be given to a competent adult if he refuses to give *consent*, even if this is life-saving treatment.
- She may ask why the blood transfusion cannot be given against his wishes by applying a section.
- Say that a section can only be applied under the Mental Health Act to patients with psychiatric problems and is not applicable in this case.
- Reassure her that the leg has stopped bleeding and as there is no clotting problem is not likely to start bleeding again, although this cannot be guaranteed. Iron therapy is likely to correct the anaemia but it is likely to happen very slowly and may take many months before it is back to normal.
- Enquire about any other concerns and answer them.
- Close the interview.

Jehovah Witnesses' beliefs about blood

Jehovah Witnesses refuse to accept blood transfusions and blood products. This includes transfusion of whole blood, packed red blood cells and plasma, as well as platelet infusion. Witnesses are also urged to discontinue their chemotherapy treatments when platelet transfusions are needed. Because Witnesses believe that any blood that leaves the body must be destroyed, they do not approve of an individual storing his own blood for a later auto-transfusion. This doctrine is based upon four passages in the Bible:

1   *Genesis 9:4* 'But flesh (meat) with . . . blood . . . ye shall not eat'
2   *Leviticus 17:12–14* '. . . No soul of you shall eat blood . . . whosoever eateth it shall be cut off'
3   *Acts 15:29* 'That ye abstain . . . from blood . . .'
4   *Acts 21:25* ' . . . Gentiles . . . keep themselves from things offered to idols and from blood . . .'.

It is important to appreciate that the decision to accept blood products is an individual one and not to be based on the assumption that all Witnesses will never accept blood transfusions. Indeed, there are dissident groups who choose to have blood, but do so anonymously as discovery may result in expulsion from their church. Hence *confidentiality* is extremely important, even with close family members.

Discussions with colleagues

Case 44: Concern about a colleague who is turning up to work drunk

Candidate information

You are a medical SHO.

Please read the scenario below. You may make notes on the paper provided. When the bell sounds enter the examination room to begin the consultation.

Subject: Dr Mark Adams

Your house officer

You have been asked to speak with your house officer, Dr Mark Adams. The ward manager has been concerned about his performance, as he has arrived at work on a number of occasions smelling of alcohol. She was particularly concerned about a recent occasion when he was asked to speak to a lady whose mother had unexpectedly died and he looked bedraggled and smelt strongly of alcohol. On another occasion one of the staff nurses had found him trying to remove drugs from the controlled drug cabinet. Your objective is to have a frank discussion with your colleague and identify any problems.

You have 14 minutes to communicate with the house doctor followed by one minute for reflection before discussion with the examiners.

Subject information

Dr Mark Adams

House officer

Dr Adams has been working as a house officer for four months now, and hates it. He particularly dislikes the long hours and resents being 'on call'. He was never keen on studying medicine and felt he was pressurised into it by his father who works as a general practitioner. He has always enjoyed a drink and finds it a good way to unwind after work. But the drinking often continues into the small hours of the morning, when he would end up in one of the city's nightclubs. It is difficult to quantify the amount of alcohol consumed, but it is not unusual to get through seven pints of beer and a few 'shorts' during the course of an evening. There have been a number of occasions when he has had no recollection of how he got home. Often in the morning he has had to have another couple of drinks to get over the terrible headaches, and then drive to work. He has been lucky not to be stopped by the police, as he is certain that he would have failed the breathalyser test. Also, of late, when possible Dr Adams would go to a pub close to the hospital for lunch, which usually included a few quick drinks. He was careful to brush his teeth and disguise his breath with mints. However, some of the nurses at work have commented that his breath smelt of alcohol, but he had told them that he had had a 'heavy night'. On one occasion he had got quite angry when one of the nurses had accused him of trying to steal drugs from the drug cabinet. He had simply been looking for paracetamol to help him with his terrible headache. He has never taken drugs and despises them.

Dr Adams himself feels that he is young and should be enjoying life to the full, and he does not think there is anything wrong with his drinking, particularly as it helps him relax and be able to speak with girls. He is not in a steady relationship at the present. His SHO has asked to speak with him and he will be horrified to hear that there are concerns about his alcohol intake and worse still, he is suspected of attempting to remove drugs from the ward. He will protest his innocence regarding the drugs charge and indeed emphasise that he is anti-drug abuse. He will also start off by denying excess alcohol consumption, but after the SHO raises concerns about patient care will accept that he probably drinks too much and agree to seek help.

Possible prompts
- I do not feel there has been a major concern with my performance.
- In all honesty I probably do not enjoy medicine as much as I should.
- Yes, I enjoy a drink and should be able to at my age. I don't feel that I drink excessively.
- On occasions I have had a drink in the morning to get over a hangover.
- I have never tried to take controlled drugs – in fact I despise drug use.
- Yes, I probably do drink excessively and should think about cutting back.

Possible interview plan
- Greet your house officer and shake his hand.
- Ask him whether he knows why you have asked to speak with him.
- If he does not know, then explain to him that there have been complaints that he may be drunk at work and also that he has been accused of trying to take controlled drugs from the cabinet.
- Listen to his response carefully, particularly trying to take note of any inconsistencies.
- Specifically enquire about any drug abuse if he has not volunteered this information thus far.
- Enquire about his alcohol consumption. Try to quantify the amount consumed. You can employ a tool such as the CAGE questionnaire, but you should remember that you are talking with a doctor and a colleague, and you must not sound patronising. It may be best to be very frank and

upfront and ask the questions directly. Ask whether he feels that he drinks excessively and whether he has ever sought help for it.

- Explain that you feel that he drinks excessively and that it is likely to affect his clinical judgement and skills. Go on to explain that because of the safety of patients and GMC guidance (see below), you will have to have a discussion with more senior staff, confidentially, which may then go on to a discussion with the GMC itself.
- You should try to be supportive and suggest that Dr Adams needs help with his alcohol consumption and advise him to get in touch with a self-help group such as Alcoholics Anonymous, Aquarius, etc.
- Thank the doctor for having this discussion and close the interview.

Good medical practice

The GMC has published excellent and relatively straightforward guidance for all registered practitioners. This is available upon request to the GMC or on their website. Points particularly pertinent to this case are numbers 26–28, shown here:

26. You must protect patients from risk of harm posed by another doctor's, or other healthcare professional's, conduct, performance or health, including problems arising from alcohol or other substance abuse. The safety of patients must come first at all times. Where there are serious concerns about a colleague's performance, health or conduct, it is essential that steps are taken without delay to investigate the concerns, to establish whether they are well-founded, and to protect patients.

27. If you have grounds to believe that a doctor or other healthcare professional may be putting patients at risk, you must give an honest explanation of your concerns to an appropriate person from the employing authority, such as the medical director, nursing director or chief executive, or the director of public health, or an officer of your local medical committee, following any procedures set by the employer. If there are no appropriate local systems, or local systems cannot resolve the problem, and you remain concerned about the safety of patients, you should inform

the relevant regulatory body. If you are not sure what to do, discuss your concerns with an impartial colleague or contact your defence body, a professional organization or the GMC for advice.

28. If you have management responsibilities you should ensure that mechanisms are in place through which colleagues can raise concerns about risks to patients.

Case 45: The hepatitis C positive doctor

Candidate information

You are a medical SHO working in a busy district general hospital.

Please read the scenario below. You may make notes on the paper provided. When the bell sounds enter the examination room to begin the consultation.

Subject: Mr Nick Stewart

Surgical SHO

This doctor who works in your hospital has asked to speak with you confidentially. He is a third-year surgical SHO, undergoing his basic surgical training. He has obtained the MRCS, and has been shortlisted for an interview leading to a training number in vascular surgery. He is extremely ambitious and career-minded. During the consultation he will tell you that about a month ago he presented to his GP with lethargy and was found to have mildly abnormal liver biochemistry. Further tests were carried out and a few days ago he found out that he is hepatitis C positive. He has not told anyone about this, but is concerned about the long-term implications and hence has contacted you today to seek some advice. Your task is to discuss his concerns with him and advise him appropriately.

You have 14 minutes to communicate with the surgical SHO followed by one minute for reflection before discussion with the examiners.

Subject information

Mr Nick Stewart

Surgical SHO

This doctor is a third-year surgical SHO about to complete his basic surgical training. He is extremely ambitious and has passed the MRCS exam and has been shortlisted for an interview leading to a specialist registrar (SpR) number in vascular surgery. His long-term ambition is to become a transplant surgeon. Approximately one month ago he saw his GP with symptoms of lethargy and was surprised to find out that his liver biochemistry was abnormal. He drinks alcohol only occasionally and swims regularly to keep fit. Further tests were carried out and a few days ago he was shocked to find out that he was hepatitis C positive. He is a heterosexual male and has never had unprotected sex, and his last sexual relationship was two years previously. Over the years he has had a few needle stick injuries (including a couple in India while on his elective) and suspects this is how he has acquired the virus. Over the past few days Mr Stewart has become increasingly anxious about his diagnosis. His concerns particularly relate to his long-term health and what effect the diagnosis may have upon his future employment prospects. In his own mind he has decided to keep the information secret from his present and future employers. However, he remains very concerned about the effect the virus will have on his own health and has decided to contact the RMO for advice. He knows that this doctor is reliable and trustworthy, and has previously worked with a hepatologist. During the course of the discussion he will inform the doctor that he does not intend to inform his employers of his diagnosis because he is afraid of the implications it will have on his employment prospects. But if the doctor is able to give good reasons, such as exposing patients to the risk of developing hepatitis C and the fact that it is a notifiable condition, Mr Stewart will consider changing his mind and agree to discuss his diagnosis with occupational health.

Possible prompts

- It came as a big surprise to find out that I was Hep C positive.
- I think I probably picked up the virus after a needle stick injury.
- I do not plan to tell any body about this, but thought it was worth getting your advice as you have worked with a hepatologist.
- Would you have to report my diagnosis to anyone?
- But I thought the information was confidential.

Possible interview plan

- Greet the doctor by name and shake his hand.
- Ask him how you can be of assistance.
- He will explain that he was recently diagnosed with hepatitis C and the sequence of events leading to it. He will elaborate and express his fears and anxieties regarding the diagnosis, particularly in relation to his future health and the implications it has upon his chosen career as a vascular surgeon, hoping to specialise as a transplant surgeon. He explains that the information that he is giving you is to be treated with the utmost confidentiality, as he does not want anyone to know that he has hepatitis C and certainly does not intend to inform his employers of his diagnosis. Remember this should be a two-way discussion with the candidate, teasing out some of this sensitive information.
- Explain to the patient that there is therapy (usually with a combination of interferon α and ribavirin) available, which can successfully eradicate the virus in up to 40–50 per cent of patients. The therapy is prolonged (up to 12 months) and does have very significant side effects. It is costly and can only be initiated by a consultant hepatologist, usually after a liver biopsy.
- Emphasise that hepatitis C is a blood-borne infection (remember that you are speaking with a professional colleague and hence very simplistic terminology as used with the lay public should not be necessary) and he potentially runs the risk of infecting patients as a surgeon. Hence it is

crucial that the hospital's occupational health team are notified, who can then advise him accordingly.

- Also hepatitis C is a notifiable condition and as such, doctors in England and Wales have a statutory duty to notify a 'proper officer' of the local authority of suspected cases (see below). All of this information needs to be relayed in a considerate and understanding manner and not in a threatening way.
- Agree on a plan to proceed. This may be agreeing to meet again in a few days to see what has transpired.
- If Mr Stewart categorically refuses to disclose his diagnosis, say that you may have to seek the advice of a senior colleague.
- Thank the subject and close.

Ethical issues

Confidentiality

Confidentiality (*see* p. 7) is extremely important in any doctor–patient relationship. When a doctor is seen as a patient, exactly the same rules apply. This includes the possible breach of the codes of confidentiality because other people may be at risk.

Doctors with infectious illness

The GMC has published excellent and relatively straightforward guidance for all registered practitioners. This is available upon request to the GMC or on their website (www.gmc-uk.org/). Points particularly pertinent to this case are shown here:

> If you know that you have a serious condition which you could pass on to patients, or that your judgment or performance could be significantly affected by a condition or illness, or its treatment, you must take and follow advice from a consultant in occupational health or another suitably qualified colleague on whether, and in what ways, you should modify your practice. Do not rely on your own assessment of the risk to patients.

> If you think you have a serious condition which you could pass on to patients, you must have all the necessary tests and act on the advice given to you by a suitably qualified colleague about necessary treatment and/or modifications to your clinical practice.

Notifiable disease

There are certain infectious conditions that doctors have a statutory duty to inform a 'proper officer' of the local authority about. The Centre for Disease Surveillance and Control (CDSC) collates this information and publishes analyses of local and national trends of these conditions. Notifiable diseases are listed here (note this list is periodically changed/added to):

- acute poliomyelitis
- anthrax
- cholera
- diphtheria
- dysentery (amoebic or bacillary)
- food poisoning (or suspected food poisoning)
- leprosy
- leptospirosis
- malaria
- measles
- meningitis
- meningococcal septicaemia (without meningitis)
- mumps
- ophthalmia neonatorum
- paratyphoid
- plague
- rabies
- relapsing fever
- rubella
- scabies
- scarlet fever
- smallpox
- tetanus
- tuberculosis
- typhoid fever
- typhus
- viral haemorrhagic fever
- viral hepatitis
- whooping cough
- yellow fever.

Case 46: The needle stick injury

Candidate information

You are on call as the RMO during a night acute medical take.

Please read the scenario below. You may make notes on the paper provided. When the bell sounds enter the examination room to begin the consultation.

Subject: Dr Alison Lucas
Medical house officer

While on a coffee break, your house officer approaches you quite upset following a needle stick injury. She explains to you that shortly after obtaining the blood from the patient, she had accidentally stabbed herself in the palm with the dirty needle. She had not been wearing gloves. Her main concern was that the patient was a vagrant, who had been admitted in a semiconscious state and was a known intravenous drug abuser. His HIV status is not known and no previous hepatitis serology is available. Your task is to counsel the house officer and to suggest any treatment that may be necessary.

You have 14 minutes to communicate with the house officer followed by one minute for reflection before discussion with the examiners. You are not required to examine the house officer.

Subject information

Dr Alison Lucas

Medical house officer

Dr Lucas has been working as a house officer for the past three months. She is a pleasant and cheerful girl, who is very conscientious and hard-working. She has been on call during the night, busy clerking patients on the medical admissions unit.

During the course of the night she saw a patient who was a vagrant and had been admitted after he was found collapsed on the street. He is a known IV drug abuser and frequently attends the accident and emergency department. She was able to elicit very little history from him, but attempted to take blood. While she was attempting to do this, the patient moved suddenly and she stabbed herself in the palm with a dirty needle. She had not been wearing any gloves at the time. She is always very cautious while taking blood and is angry with herself for not wearing gloves, which she normally does. Now she is very worried about the possibility of having contracted an infection from him, particularly as he is an IV drug abuser. HIV is of particular concern, but she is also worried about hepatitis, although she knows she has been immunised to hepatitis B. Upon checking the man's medical records, there is no documentation of any previous serological tests. She decides to have a discussion with her SHO (the candidate) and ask them if they can carry out an HIV test on the patient and whether she needs any prophylactic treatment.

Possible prompts
- What is the chance of me developing HIV?
- What is the chance of me developing hepatitis?
- Do I need prophylactic treatment?
- Can we do an HIV test on him?
- Will I have to take time off work?

Possible interview plan
- Greet the doctor and ask her how you can help her.
- She will tell you about her needle stick injury and the circumstances in which it happened. The person she received the injury from is a vagrant who is known to be an IV drug abuser. She will go on to tell you that she is very concerned about the possibility of an infective illness, particularly HIV.
- Ask whether she was wearing gloves at the time and ensure that she has been immunised to hepatitis B. She will tell you

that she wasn't wearing gloves, but is immunised to hepatitis B.

- Also ask how much blood there was on the needle before she stabbed herself with it.
- Explain to her that the risk of transmission of infectious disease through a needle stick injury is significant, but small, and depends on numerous factors such as the amount of blood on the dirty needle, depth of penetration, etc. Generally speaking the risk of transmission of hepatitis C is 3 per cent and HIV is 0.3 per cent. Hepatitis B is the greatest risk at 30 per cent, but she will be immune to this.
- Say that you will discuss the case with the microbiologist/ infectious disease consultant on call to decide whether she requires post-exposure prophylaxis (PEP – see below) to reduce the chances of her acquiring HIV.
- And advise her to inform occupational health of the incident. Baseline bloods need to be taken and then bloods at 3 and 6 months to look for seroconversion. If they remain negative, she can be given the all clear. She will also have to have her hepatitis B and C serology checked.
- She may go on to suggest that maybe we should take blood from the patient to check for the presence of these infections and that she would be reassured if these came back negative. Tell her that this is not possible, without prior consent and counselling of the patient. But when he wakes up you will discuss this with him (reassure her that the discussions will be strictly confidential and see if he agrees).
- Ask her to look out for signs of acute hepatitis, particularly jaundice, and be vigilant to symptoms suggestive of a seroconversion illness. These include fevers, malaise, lethargy, rashes and enlarged lymph nodes.
- Remind her that, while the risk is small, there is a possibility of her carrying an infectious illness and it would be prudent to use a barrier form of contraception until she can be sure that she is not infected.
- Reassure her that many, if not most, doctors have a needle stick injury during the course of their careers and the risk of acquiring serious illness is extremely small.

- Ask her if she has any other concerns or questions and whether she feels well enough to carry on with her work.
- If she can continue and has no further concerns, close the interview.

Needle stick injuries

The rates of transmission of blood-borne viruses vary, but generally speaking can be remembered by the rule of 3s:

- *hepatitis B* is 30 per cent (if the source patient is highly infectious)
- *hepatitis C* is 3 per cent
- *HIV* is 0.3 per cent.

HIV tends to cause the most anxiety among healthcare professionals (and indeed the lay public who are injured by discarded needles), but hepatitis B and hepatitis C are more infectious. Several factors are significant in the transmission from an infected source. These include:

- the depth of the injury and size of the needle
- the level of contamination of the sharp
- the site of the injury, e.g. higher risk if straight into a blood vessel
- the 'infectiousness' or viral load of the source patient.

Where the source patient is known, it is imperative that their consent is obtained before testing for their hepatitis and HIV status. This point is made very clear in the GMC guidance on serious communicable disease.

Post-exposure prophylaxis (PEP)

Where individuals have been exposed to hepatitis B or HIV, the possibility of post exposure prophylaxis should be considered as soon as possible.

- In the non-immune subject, prophylaxis for *hepatitis B* is hyper immune gamma globulin. This should be administered as soon as possible and followed up by an accelerated course of hepatitis B vaccination.

- Where the donor is known to be *HIV* positive, prophylaxis should be commenced as soon as possible and preferably within the hour. For this reason, many hospital accident and emergency departments carry a kit for rapid access. The drugs generally used include a cocktail of zidovudine, lamivudine and indinavir. These have to be taken for 28 days and may cause severe side effects such as nausea and lethargy, which may mean that the doctor is unable to work.
- Currently there is no recommended post-exposure prophylaxis following potential hepatitis C exposures. However, there is data that shows that if acute hepatitis C infection is confirmed in the exposed person, early treatment with alpha interferon may be highly effective in preventing the development of chronic hepatitis C infection.

Other issues
- Confidentiality (*see* p. 7).
- Counselling for a HIV test (*see* case 20).

Case 47: Bullying

Candidate information

You are a cardiology SHO working on a busy CCU.

Please read the scenario below. You may make notes on the paper provided. When the bell sounds enter the examination room to begin the consultation.

Subject: Dr Amanda Walters

House officer

Dr Walters has been working as your house officer for the past three months. She previously worked as an ENT house officer and had a great time, but is really finding it tough in her current post, even though she has aspirations of becoming a cardiologist. She has asked to meet up with you to discuss her difficulties. During the discussion she tells you that she feels that she is being bullied by the registrar, who belittles her at every opportunity and on occasions has made remarks in public that she found extremely offensive: he had joked with the nursing staff that it wasn't too late for her to become a nurse as the patients would always assume that she was a nurse anyway. On another occasion he had suggested that she should try wearing shorter skirts if she wanted to get ahead. The consultant she works for is very approachable, but is rarely on the CCU. Moreover, he is very friendly with the registrar and Dr Walters is concerned that complaining may have negative repercussions for her career. Hence she has chosen to consult you for advice. Your task is to listen to her concerns and give her appropriate advice.

You have 14 minutes to communicate with the house officer followed by one minute for reflection before discussion with the examiners.

Subject information

Dr Amanda Walters

House officer

Dr Walters has been working in her current post as a cardiology PRHO for three months and is finding it very difficult. This is despite the fact that she wants to specialise as a cardiologist. The main reason for her difficulties is her registrar, who constantly belittles her opinion and has even made offensive remarks about her in public. On one occasion he had joked with the CCU nurses that it wasn't too late for Dr Walters to retrain as a nurse as patients would always assume she was a nurse anyway. Worse still, he had on an occasion suggested that she should wear shorter skirts if she wanted to get ahead in cardiology. There have been numerous other comments and Dr Walters is finding it difficult to cope with it now. She has always prided herself on being hard-working, diligent and having the ability to get along with every one. Indeed, she had excelled as an ENT house officer before commencing this present post. Dr Walters does not want to come across as a whiner and is reluctant to approach the consultant, who is friendly and approachable, but rarely on the ward and also seems to be on very friendly terms with the registrar. Hence she is concerned that this could have negative repercussions for her career aspirations. Instead she has chosen to speak with her senior house officer who will advise her accordingly.

Possible prompts
- I'm not happy in this post.
- The registrar often belittles me in front of others.
- He has made many inappropriate comments.
- I'm concerned that if I complain it will affect my career.

Possible interview plan
- Greet the doctor and shake hands with her
- Set the agenda. Ask her how you can help her.
- Listen to her concerns in a non-judgemental manner. She

will tell you that she is finding her current post difficult and attributes this to the registrar, who belittles her and has made inappropriate remarks.

- Say that this is a very serious matter and ask if she is absolutely confident that this is not a simple misunderstanding.
- Ask whether she has provoked this behaviour in any way. She will tell you she has not.
- Ask her if anyone else had noticed his animosity towards her and if she knew of other members of staff who had been similarly aggrieved by his attitude.
- Explain to her that this behaviour is inappropriate and that she should not have to put up with it and ask her (if she has not already volunteered the information) if she has any reservations about relaying this information to the consultant. She will tell you that she is concerned about the potentially negative effect this may have on her career.
- Ask her if she would mind you speaking with the consultant.
- If she does not mind then tell her that you will take the matter up with the consultant, who can then decide whether it is a disciplinary matter.
- If she does not want you to speak with the consultant, then explain to her that you can anonymously discuss the matter with another consultant or the medical director. Alternatively, the British Medical Association can be approached for advice.
- Also tell her that there are excellent anonymous counselling services available for doctors and you can obtain a contact number for her if she feels that she is having difficulty coping.
- Tell her that you will contact her once you have had the opportunity to discuss the matter with a consultant.
- Ask her if she has any other questions or concerns.
- If she does not, close the interview.

Bullying and harassment

Junior doctors are particularly prone to bullying and harassment in the workplace. One study (Quine, 1999) found that 37 per cent of junior doctors had experienced some form of bullying within the previous year. Of greatest risk were female doctors and those from the ethnic minorities. Bullying is defined in terms of its negative effect on the recipient and not the intention of the protagonist. The behaviour has to be persistent and it can affect the victim in a number of different ways (Rayner and Hoel, 1997):

- threats to professional status (e.g. belittling opinion, public humiliation)
- threats to personal standing (e.g. insults, teasing)
- isolation (e.g. withholding information)
- overwork (e.g. impossible deadlines)
- destabilisation (e.g. meaningless tasks).

In the UK there is no specific law in relation to bullying, but cases are tried under related laws such as personal/psychiatric injury, breach of contract, negligence and even manslaughter, where bullying led to suicide.

The GMC, in its good practice guidelines, makes it clear that you must always treat your colleagues fairly and in particular must not discriminate against colleagues on grounds of their sex, race or disability. Moreover, the guidelines go on to say that a doctor must not allow their views of colleagues' lifestyle, culture, beliefs, colour, gender, sexuality, or age to prejudice their professional relationship with them.

References

Quine, L (1999) Workplace bullying in an NHS community trust: staff questionnaire survey. *BMJ*. **318**: 228–32.

Rayner C and Hoel H (1997) A summary review of literature relating to workplace bullying. *J Comm Appl Soc Psychol*. **7**: 181–91.

Case 48: The distressed medical student

Candidate information

You are the SHO working on the intensive care unit.

Please read the scenario below. You may make notes on the paper provided. When the bell sounds enter the examination room to begin the consultation.

Subject: Miss Elaine Mayfield

Medical student

This 21-year-old medical student has been on an 'attachment' on the ITU for the past three weeks. This is one of her first clinical attachments and over the past three weeks she has spent much of her time looking after Mrs Sandra Micheals, who was admitted to the ITU after she had developed severe septicaemia. Since admission she has made good progress and was extubated a few days ago. Both the medical team and her family were optimistic that she would be well enough to be discharged from the unit, before too long. However, during the previous night she deteriorated suddenly and despite the best efforts of the ITU team, died from a presumed pulmonary embolus. The following morning, Elaine Mayfield is extremely distressed by her sudden death and has spent a considerable amount of time crying in the sister's office. The sister has been trying to console her, and has now asked you to speak with the young student to reassure her that nothing else could have been done.

You have 14 minutes to communicate with the medical student followed by one minute for reflection before discussion with the examiners.

Subject information

Miss Elaine Mayfield

Medical student

This 24-year-old medical student has been attached to the ITU for the past three weeks. This is only her second clinical attachment, the first one being with a general practitioner. During her time on the ITU the student has spent much of her time helping to look after Mrs Sandra Micheals. This 28-year-old lady had been admitted to the ITU after she had developed severe septicaemia, which required aggressive management with anti-biotics, inotropic and ventilatory support. Since her admission to the ITU, Mrs Micheals had been making a slow and steady recovery and had been extubated a few days ago. Both the medical team and her family were optimistic that she would be well enough to be discharged from the ITU before too long. Her family consisted of her husband and two children aged two and four years. Her parents and two sisters were also very devoted and visited regularly. Over the weeks the student had developed a close bond with the family. However, one morning she arrived to find Mrs Micheals bed was vacant and she was very distressed to find out that during the night she had suddenly deteriorated and died. Elaine has never previously had to deal with death either of a patient or relative, and her inability to deal with it has come as a real shock. The sister on the ITU had been very supportive and had asked her to sit in the office until she felt better and had also asked one of the doctors working on the ITU (the candidate) to have a chat with her to reassure her further and to explain that little could have been done to change the outcome. The chat will help and Elaine will feel much better at the end of it.

Possible prompts

- I'm finding it very difficult to cope with Mrs Micheals' death.
- It was so sudden.
- I should be grown up about it.

- It will be impossible for me to work as a doctor if I break down every time I lose a patient.
- Speaking about it does seem to help.

Possible interview plan

- Greet the student and shake hands with her.
- Set the agenda. Explain to her that the sister has asked you to speak with her about the death of Mrs Micheals. Ask if she minds talking about it.
- Ask if she has ever had to deal with the death of anyone previously. She will tell you she has not.
- Now go into the reasons for her being so upset.
- Let her speak at her own pace with you giving prompts:
  - 'Was it the sudden nature of Mrs Micheals' death?'
  - 'Do you feel the death could have been prevented?'
  - 'Do you feel that you were overattached to the patient?'
- Tell her that while this patient's death was sudden and unexpected, it is unlikely that anything could have been done to prevent it.
- In sympathetic terms, remind her that death is the natural end to life and is something that we have to regularly confront during the course of our medical practices. Often death is totally unexpected and seemingly unfair.
- With time no doubt we get better at developing coping mechanisms. However, we are not only doctors, but also human and often let personal feelings creep into our work. This is OK and can make us more caring doctors.
- Ask gently if speaking about the death of this patient is making it easier for her. Tell her that talking about the death will help her come to terms with it.
- Follow up. Tell her that you will speak with her again in a few days' time and see how she is getting on. Remind her that there are counselling services available through her GP and through the university and if she has difficulty coping long term, she should seek help early.
- Close the interview.

Ethical issues

Loss of someone (particularly sudden and unexpected loss) leads to grief reactions and the bereavement process. Doctors and other healthcare professionals are not immune to this process. *See* p. 155 for further discussion on bereavement.

Support for the doctor

As part of their workload, doctors are constantly forming emotional relationships with patients and their families, and are then exposed to their helplessness, suffering, uncertainty, occasionally anger and death. This can have profound long-term effects on the doctor's well-being leading to depression, substance abuse and even suicide.

Regrettably, the culture of the health service in the UK (and perhaps most parts of the world) has been such that healthcare professionals found it difficult to express personal emotions regarding the death of patients. It was seen as a weakness and the difficulty in coping may have implications on a career within the hierarchical structure of the NHS. Personal observation suggests that doctors are much worse at dealing with the death of patients than nurses, who tend to talk about and often mourn the loss of a patient. Fortunately, the climate does seem to be changing and both individual doctors and the trusts they work for are becoming more aware of the stressful nature of our work, and help in terms of either counselling or an informal chat with a colleague is not frowned upon these days.

Case 49: The near miss: discussion with the nurse

(Review this case with case 30: The near miss: discussion with patient)

Candidate information

You are a medical SHO working on a chest ward.

Please read the scenario below. You may make notes on the paper provided. When the bell sounds enter the examination room to begin the consultation.

Subject: staff nurse Jo Nesbitt

Age: 28 years

Re: Mr John Powell, aged 39 years

You have decided to speak with this nurse after the patient had complained that she had made a potentially life-threatening error. The patient is a 39-year-old man who was admitted following a severe attack of asthma and had been commenced on prednisolone. He was known to have a severe allergy to aspirin and had previously been admitted to the ITU after ingestion of aspirin. He has alleged that during the morning drug round the nurse had got her prescription sheets mixed up and given him aspirin, which was intended for the patient in the next bed. He had spotted the mistake just before taking the tablets and had been very upset by the incident. Your objective is to have a discussion with the staff nurse involved to hear her side of the story and to devise an action plan.

You have 14 minutes to communicate with the staff nurse followed by one minute for reflection before discussion with the examiners.

Subject information

Staff nurse Jo Nesbitt

Aged 28 years

Re: Mr John Powell, aged 39 years

The SHO working on the medical ward has asked to speak with this nurse regarding an incident earlier in the day. She had been giving out medication during the drug round and had given Mr John Powell aspirin instead of his prescription, which was prednisolone. Mr Powell, who is a 39-year-old asthmatic, had spotted the mistake and was very angry with the nurse and had threatened to make an official complaint. He is known to have a severe allergy to aspirin, which had previously resulted in an ITU admission. The nurse had acknowledged her mistake and had apologised immediately, but she had not been able to calm him down and the sister on the ward had to intervene. This episode had been very upsetting for the young nurse, who normally prides herself on her caution and can only attribute her mistake to the fact that her mind has been preoccupied with personal matters. She has been very depressed of late because of her father, who has recently been diagnosed with terminal cancer, and the break-up of a long-term relationship with her boyfriend, who had 'dumped' her. When she speaks with the doctor, SN Nesbitt will not hesitate in admitting her mistake and will attribute her mistake to her own difficult personal life.

Possible prompts

- Yes, I gave the wrong medication to the patient.
- No, I had not checked his identity and I didn't realise he was allergic to aspirin.
- I'm having a lot of personal problems of late and am finding it difficult to concentrate on the job.

Possible interview plan

- Greet the nurse.
- Set the agenda. Tell her that you need to speak with her

regarding an incident where a patient claimed that he had been given the wrong medication.

- Ask her to tell you about the incident. She will honestly tell you that a patient had been given aspirins by mistake, but had noticed the error and not taken them.
- Check whether she had verified the patient's identification before giving him the drug and whether she was aware that the patient who had been given aspirin was severely allergic to this drug. She will reply in the negative to both of these points.
- Ask her to tell you why this mistake occurred and how it could have been prevented. She may tell you that she has a lot of personal problems, which are affecting her ability to work.
- Tell the nurse that this was potentially a very serious mistake and it is important that an incident form is completed to ensure that steps are taken to prevent it happening again. For the same reason it is important that the sister in charge of the ward and the consultant looking after the patient are informed, particularly as the patient is likely to complain to them.
- Regarding her personal problems, tell her that she should seek help through her GP and occupational health. She may need time off work or perhaps only carry out low-risk tasks for a while.
- Reassure her that the purpose of any future investigation is not to look for evidence to incriminate her, but to review practice on the ward to prevent a similar mistake happening again.
- Summarise the discussion and close the interview.

Important issues

Review case 30 (p. 131) and the brief discussion on clinical governance.

> 'Accidents hardly ever happen without warning. The combination or sequence of failures and mistakes that causes an accident may indeed be unique, but the individual failures and mistakes rarely are.'
>
> (Mike O'Leary (British Airways, UK), Sheryl Chappell (NASA, United States))

Case 50: The offensive doctor

Candidate information

You are an SHO working on a care of the elderly ward.

Please read the scenario below. You may make notes on the paper provided. When the bell sounds enter the examination room to begin the consultation.

Subject: Dr Robert Ling

Your house officer

You have been asked to speak with your house officer, Dr Robert Ling, because of an outburst recently. The sister on the ward was very concerned when Dr Ling lost his temper and shouted at the nursing staff. The sister has told you that the young doctor is generally unapproachable and often rude. In particular, she is concerned about an episode where he was asked to catheterise an elderly male patient and he had refused point-blank, saying that he didn't catheterise stinking patients and the nurses should be sufficiently trained to carry out such duties. Unfortunately there hadn't been a trained nurse to carry out the catheterisation and the man had been left in agony with urinary obstruction before another doctor could be found to carry out the task. You have arranged to speak with the doctor about the sister's concerns.

You have 14 minutes to communicate with the doctor followed by one minute for reflection before discussion with the examiners.

Subject information

Dr Robert Ling

House officer

Dr Ling has been working as a house officer for nine weeks on the care of the elderly ward. He was an outstanding student at medical school, regularly achieving distinctions. Towards the end of his training he became certain that he did not enjoy clinical medicine and decided to have a career in either academic medicine or perhaps leave medicine altogether and go into an alternative vocation. His parents had been extremely proud of him becoming a doctor and he is worried about what effect him changing career will have on them. Working as a house officer has confirmed his resolution, and as each day goes by he is finding the task more difficult to cope with. He is unhappy about the hours he has to work and the demoralising conditions of the ward and he feels unappreciated as a junior doctor. He particularly dislikes clinical tasks and although he does not usually lose his temper, was unable to control himself when one of the nurses had asked him to catheterise a patient. He has always understood this to be a nursing duty and had no intention of performing the task. The nurse had become very upset and he was half expecting today's discussion with his senior house officer. During the discussion, Dr Ling will be honest about his difficulties with clinical medicine and his plan to either go into academic medicine or leave the profession altogether. He will listen to and accept his colleague's advice.

Possible prompts

- Yes, I was asked to catheterise a patient, but refused to do this as I felt this was a nursing duty.
- I feel that I don't enjoy clinical medicine and am thinking about changing my career. Perhaps go into academic medicine or leave the profession all together.

Possible interview plan

- Greet your house officer.

- Ask him whether he knows why you have asked to speak with him.
- If he does not know then explain to him that there have been complaints that he has been unapproachable and refused to catheterise a man who was left in agony for a number of hours.
- Ask him to relay his version of the incident. He is likely to tell you that he was indeed asked to catheterise the man, but he felt it was an inappropriate duty and one that nurses should perform.
- Tell him you disagree on this point. Say that the duties of doctors and nurses often overlap, depending upon the training of the staff involved. The problem here is that there were no trained nurses and a patient was left to suffer, and the urinary retention could potentially cause irreversible damage.
- Move on to the complaints about his general behaviour and ask him whether he felt there was a problem.
- At this point he may tell you that he is unhappy working as a house officer and is thinking about an alternative career. In particular he will say that he feels that he has poor working conditions and feels unappreciated as a doctor.
- Say that you respect his views and working as a doctor can be very challenging at times. Working conditions are often difficult, but there seems to be a real push to improve them, and perhaps he hasn't been in the job long enough to develop a broader picture (you must not sound patronising at this point).
- What's more, medicine is a very diverse speciality and most people find a niche within it. He may choose to disagree with you on this point.
- Say that he needs to speak with his clinical supervisor about his future career and the options open to him. But while he is working as a doctor, it is very important that he does not do the task half-heartedly, which may potentially endanger patients. Tell him that as his SHO you will help and support him to the best of your abilities.
- Ask him if there are any other issues he would like to discuss.
- If not, thank him and close the interview.

Appendices

Appendix 1: Driving and disease

(www.dvla.gov.uk/at_a_glance/content.htm)

	Group 1	Group 2
MI	4-week ban	6-week ban
Epilepsy	1-year ban/Can only restart driving if fit-free or only has fit during sleep	10-year ban
Diabetes	OK if there are no hypos	Banned if on insulin or there are visual problems
TIA	1-month ban	1-year ban
CVA	1-month ban	5-year ban

Appendix 2: Marksheet

ROYAL COLLEGES OF PHYSICIANS OF THE UNITED KINGDOM
MRCP(UK) PACES EXAMINATION - CLINICAL MARKSHEET
STATION FOUR: Communication Skills and Ethics

CANDIDATE NAME (PLEASE PRINT)

Examination Number

Centre Number

Sheet No. 6

Examiners are required to make a judgement of the candidate's performance in each of the sections (1, 2 and 3) by filling in the appropriate box like this ━. Please use 2B pencil only.

Brief description of case:

Examiner Number:

EXAMINER
(PLEASE PRINT NAME AND SIGN BELOW)

	clear pass	pass	fail	clear fail
1. Communication Skills - Conduct of Interview • Introduces self to patient and explains role clearly • Agrees the purpose of the interview with the patient • Puts the patient at ease and establishes good rapport • Explores the patient's concerns, feelings and expectations - demonstrates empathy, respect and non-judgemental attitude • Prioritises problems and redirects interview sensitively	▭	▭	▭	▭
2. Communication Skills - exploration and problem negotiation • Appropriate questioning style - generally open-ended to closed as the interview progresses • Provides clear explanations (jargon-free) that the patient understands • Agrees a clear course of action • Summarises and checks the patient's understanding • Concludes the interview appropriately	▭	▭	▭	▭
3. Ethics and Law In relation to the clinical scenario the candidate demonstrates knowledge of the relevant ethical and legal principles and appropriate attitudes in making decisions • Knowledge of ethical principles • Understanding legal constraints applicable to case • Provides adequate reasoning as appropriate to case	▭	▭	▭	▭

Now record your overall judgement of the candidate's performance taking into account the above: please grade as clear pass/pass/fail/ clear fail, (a fail or clear fail grade must be accompanied by clearly written explanatory comments).

Counselling Recommended ▭

COMMENTS (PLEASE PRINT)

overall judgement

clear pass	pass	fail	clear fail
▭	▭	▭	▭

please continue in the unshaded area overleaf in necessary

Useful web pages

Action on Smoking and Health (ASH):	www.ash.org.uk/
Asthma UK:	www.asthma.org.uk/
BMA:	web.bma.org.uk/
BMA ethics:	www.bma.org.uk/public/ethics.nsf/
British Liver Trust:	www.britishlivertrust.org.uk/ content/home/default.asp
Cancer bacup:	www.cancerbacup.org.uk/Home
Department of Health:	www.doh.gov.uk
Diabetes UK:	www.diabetes.org.uk/
Down's syndrome Association:	www.downs-syndrome.org.uk/
DVLA:	www.dvla.gov.uk/
DVLA (at a glance):	www.dvla.gov.uk/at a glance/content.htm
Ethnicity:	www.ethnicityonline.net/default.htm
Epilepsy Action:	www.epilepsy.org.uk/
General Medical Council (GMC):	www.gmc-uk.org/
International Huntington Association:	www.huntington-assoc.com/
Macmillan cancer relief:	www.macmillan.org.uk/
MRCP (UK):	www.mrcpuk.org/index2.html
MS Society:	www.mssociety.org.uk/
National Association for Crohn's and Colitis (NACC):	www.nacc.org.uk/
National Institute for Clinical Excellence (NICE):	www.nice.org.uk
Parkinson's disease:	www.parkinsons.org.uk/HomePage. asp?NodeID=89586
Resuscitation Council:	www.resus.org.uk
Terrence Higgins Trust:	www.tht.org.uk/
UK Transplant:	www.uktransplant.org.uk/ukt/default.jsp

Index

Page numbers in italic refer to landmark cases

Printed in Great Britain
by Amazon.co.uk, Ltd.,
Marston Gate.